Illustrations of the
Complete Acupuncture System:
the Sinew, Luo, Divergent,
Eight Extraordinary and Primary Channels

Disclaimer and Note: The information presented in this book relates to the subject of what is known in the Eastern
Medical Community as "Traditional Chinese Medicine" and "Classical Chinese Medicine" and is intended solely for
the use by Licensed Acupuncturists and students under the supervised study of acupuncture through an accredited
educational institution. Under no circumstances is the information in this work to be used or acted upon by an
unlicensed, untrained or unsupervised individual. The Author and Publisher do not advocate or endorse self-diagnosis,
self-medication or treatment by unlicensed individuals under any circumstances. Chinese Medicine is a regulated
profession and subject to the jurisdiction of the individual states as well as local and national professional and
accrediting organizations. Individuals are strongly encouraged to perform their own due diligence and seek guidance
and referrals from these organizations or other licensed professionals.

The basis of the teachings in this book come from the oral tradition through the gracious generosity of my principal
teacher, Daoist Master, Dr. Jeffrey Yuen. I have made interpretations, extrapolations, connections, additions, orderings
and constructed all the protocols contained in this book and in the book Advanced Acupuncture, A Clinic Manual.
This book contains contributions from my clinical practice. Any mistakes are mine. A.C.S.

Illustrations: Pat Didner
Cover design, book design, graphic design: Cody Dodo
Front cover calligraphy: "The gentle rains of heaven cleanse us of our illnesses."
Gift of Dr. Jeffrey Yuen to the Classical Wellness Center, 2008.
ISBN: 978-0-9837720-3-3

Illustrations of the Complete Acupuncture System:

the Sinew, Luo, Divergent, Eight Extraordinary and Primary Channels

A Companion to
Advanced Acupuncture
A Clinic Manual

Ann Cecil-Sterman

Illustrations by Pat Didner

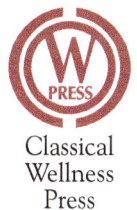

Classical
Wellness
Press

Contents

The Eight Extraordinary Channels   46

The Primary Channels   64

Author's Note

This publication is a response to countless requests for a separate collection of the drawings that appear in the book *Advanced Acupuncture, A Clinic Manual*, the first book of protocols for the Complement Channels.

Taken together, these drawings map the entire channel system comprising the Complement Channels—the Sinew, Luo, Divergent and Eight Extraordinary channels—and the Primary Channels. I am hoping that this easy form of reference will be helpful in the clinic when there is not enough time to thumb through the heavy, red book. Concepts and principles being understood, there are times when a quick reference secures confidence and precision. Out of respect for this complex material, I have omitted all instruction and the treatment protocols.

May your use of the Complement Channels expand more readily with this additional tool.

Thank you for being a part of the expanding, world-wide cultivation and use of these remarkable channels as our profession returns to the rich and precious roots of our medicine as described in the Han Dynasty texts, the foundation of Chinese Medicine.

The oral transmission that traditionally has accompanied transmission of the difficult classical texts of Chinese medicine is the light that elucidates and inspires. I am deeply grateful for the gracious generosity of my teacher Daoist Master, Dr Jeffrey Yuen, the 88th generation of his Taoist lineage: Yu Ching Huang Lao Pai, (Jade PuritySchool, Yellow Emperor/Lao Tzu sect); 26th generation of Chuan Chen Lung Men Pai (Complete Reality School, Dragon Gate Sect).

The transmissions I have received have come through my filter; any mistakes are mine.

With warm wishes,
Ann

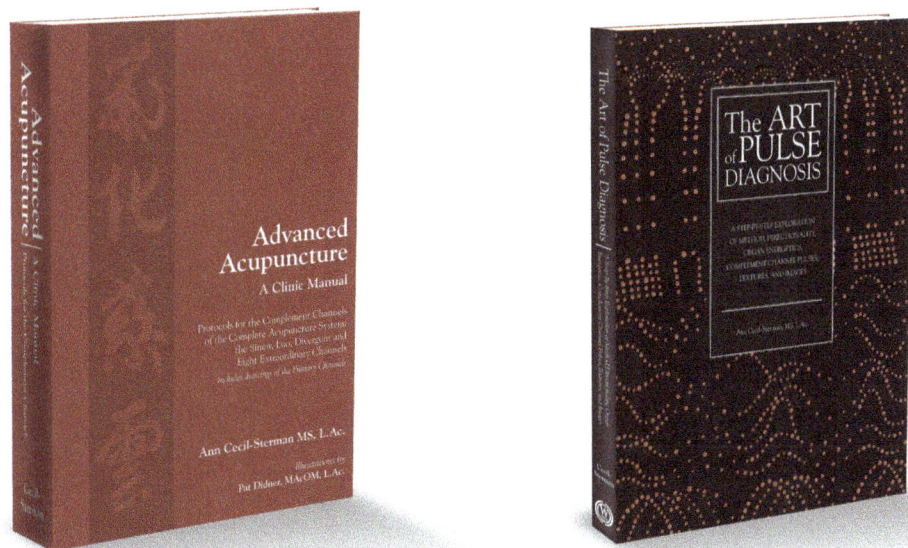

A Note on the Illustrations

Four years before the Clinic Manual (2013) was published, I sent out a group email asking whether there was an acupuncturist out there who also happened to be an artist. That same day, I received a reply from my colleague (and now good friend) Pat Didner. She shared excitement about the project, understood its importance and was soon at work.

The illustrations took three years to complete. Pat has an amazing and quick eye and a ready and deep intuitive sense. I'm certain the Manual would not have been possible without her. The Primary and Complement Channels are extremely complex and there were many aspects to consider during the countless hours of discussions between us. Pat developed a unique way of conveying vital information and the result is deeply meaningful and beautiful. The most wonderful thing to me is that the drawings truly are art.

We decided to put nearly every channel on a separate page as a way of showing that the tiniest and simplest channel is just as important as the longest one with the most branches.

These drawings present some information about the channels that had not been shown before the Manual was published. The Sinew Channels, for example, are shown with their actual width, that is, covering the entire surface of the body and overlapping with one another. Pat has achieved this beautifully, devising a way to show the real width and complexity of the Sinews and the clarity of the bindings without losing the definition of the trajectories. The organs are generally not shown in the drawings for the simple reason that when the Classical texts refer to the treatment of an organ, they are referring to a point that has access to that organ since the organs themselves cannot be directly needled. The Mu and Shu points have this function and they are shown in order to facilitate visualization of the completed treatment and its connection with the viscera.

We felt the manual would not be complete without a set of illustrations of the Primary Channels drawn according to the descriptions in the Classical texts. Although the focus here is not on Primary Channel theory or practice, the inclusion of the Primary Channels drawn this way will also help in determining Transverse Luo and Emptied Luo diagnoses.

About the Author

Ann Cecil-Sterman, MS, L.Ac, is the author of widely acclaimed book, *Advanced Acupuncture: A Clinic Manual*, a required text in many acupuncture schools in the United States, Europe and Australia. She travels all over the world, to Spain, England, Italy, Canada, Australia, Belgium, Mexico and all over the United States to teach the application and methodology of the Complement Channels, the art of pulse diagnosis, and the use of food as medicine. For many years she taught Advanced Clinical Observation and was a senior clinic supervisor at the school of acupuncture founded by Dr Jeffrey Yuen in 1997 in New York City. She is a long-time student of Dr Yuen, having extensively studied acupuncture, diet, Chinese medical history, herbs, qigong, essential oils, stones and philosophy with him across North America. Ann's practice features the Complement Channels of acupuncture: the Sinew, Luo, Divergent and Eight Extraordinary Channels, and is augmented with Classical Chinese dietary therapeutic guidance. Currently, her patients—children and adults of all ages come from all over the world, working through illnesses or on personal cultivation. She lives in Manhattan with her husband and two children. Her most recent book, *The Art of Pulse Diagnosis*, is widely in use.

About the Illustrator

Pat Didner, MAcOM, L.Ac, is an acupuncturist board certified in Chinese herbal medicine and a graduate of the Academy of Oriental Medicine at Austin Graduate School of Integrative Medicine. She has done extensive Asian bodywork training in tui na with Yongxin Fan as well as training in Qigong Anma with Devon Hornby. A long-time practitioner of tai chi and qigong, Pat continues training with Sifu Fong Ha and studies Classical Chinese Medicine with Ann-Cecil Sterman. Pat specializes in the treatment of chronic conditions, pain, emotional and stress-related concerns, family and women's health, including infertility, using acupuncture, bodywork, Chinese herbal medicine and nutritional counseling. Pat has an art and art history background and enjoys drawing. She lives with her family and practices in New York City.

About the Designer

Cody Dodo, MS, L.Ac, studied acupuncture under Dr Jeffrey Yuen at the Swedish Institute in New York and later completed advanced studies with Dr Yuen in acupuncture and Chinese dietary therapy. Prior to his pursuit of acupuncture, Cody had a long career as a graphic designer in the publishing industry. He also designed the author's first book, *Advanced Acupuncture: A Clinic Manual*. Cody has a private practice in Manhattan, teaches Classical Acupuncture internationally, and lives with his wife in Brooklyn.

Acknowledgments

Thank you so much Pat Didner, Cody Dodo, Andrew Sterman, Hope Hathaway and Gabrielle Zlotnik.

The Importance of the Complete Acupuncture System

The *Nei Jing* explains the Complete Acupuncture System of Channels and Collaterals, a vast system comprising five classes of channel: Sinew, Primary, Luo, Divergent and Eight Extraordinary. The Primary Channels are responsible for the minute-to-minute functioning of the organs. The other channels—known collectively as the Complement Channels—provide the remainder of the complete energetic picture of the body; in the presence of pathology the Complement Channels allow the uninterrupted functioning of the Primary Channels. The Sinews, Luos and Divergents move pathology into and out of latency ensuring the preservation of life through their often complex mechanisms. The Eight Extraordinary Channels allow life to unfold to its full potential while also absorbing pathology that has entered the Yuan level.

The Complement Channels have no limit to their application, and are the channels that the acupuncturist can use to understand and then to reverse the course of chronic degenerative diseases. They are the key to a detailed understanding of how the body deals with a pathological encounter that it was unable to fully handle at the time of invasion. They explain the mechanisms that protect the viscera during the progression of disease. The Complement Channels are also a model for understanding (and even altering) personal evolution, including our personal emotional journey and its impact on our physiology.

The human body recognizes that the disease of an internal organ is the most serious of all illnesses. Using very sophisticated strategies (described by the Complement Channels), the body shifts a pathogen out of the Primary Channels to ensure the safety of the organs, or in the case of the Sinew Channels, prevents penetration of the Primary Channels altogether. In the presence of a potentially life-threatening disease the Complement Channels move the illness away from the Zang Fu, creating a different disease so that the viscera are less immediately threatened; they shift an acute condition into latency or they create "slower" disease. The Complement Channels are present literally to preserve humanity.

A practitioner of these channels, through the examination of pulses, tongue and palpation, determines which channel is being employed to keep the pathogen at bay and then decides whether the body needs more help to do so (accentuating the body's command of the channel in its suppressive capacity), or whether it's time to give the body a directive to expel the pathogen (encouraging the body to engage the channel in its releasing capacity), or to move the pathogen to a different channel altogether.

The Complement Channels are utterly necessary for a complete understanding of the energetics of the full acupuncture system and its clinical application. This set of illustrations is a companion to my book, Advanced Acupuncture, A Clinic Manual which explores the importance of the Complement Channels and offers theory and treatment protocols for every acupuncture channel, considering all five classes of channel of equal importance in the Complete System of Acupuncture.

Interrelationships of the Complete Acupuncture System

The Complement Channels perform the common function of keeping pathology away from the Zang Fu. A pathogen will first encounter the Sinew Channels which create sneezes, sweat, coughing, vomiting, diarrhea or frequent urination to release the pathogen. They can also create tightness to hold the pathogen in the exterior until enough resources have been gathered to release it.

Aspects of Latency of a Pathogenic Factor

1 If the Sinews fail, the pathogen moves either to the Divergent or to the Luo Channels. When those avenues are exhausted, the Eight Extra Channels can absorb the pathology. When a pathogen is being held latent in the Luos, Divergents or Eight Extras, there are no signs or symptoms.

2 If the Tai Yang Sinew—the very first line of defense for an external pathogenic factor—fails and the Luo Channels do not absorb the pathogen, the pathogen can enter the He-Sea point of the Bladder Primary Channel. The body diverts the pathogen from the Bladder organ (to which the He-Sea has access) to the joints. The pathogen has entered the Divergent Channel sequence at that point.

3 If the Luo Channels are taxed due to Ying (Blood or Fluid) deficiency, the pathogen can go to the Divergent Channels.

4 If the Sinews fail due to insufficient Yang, the pathogen can go to the joints. As Jing declines, latency is lost (symptoms emerge as the pathogen becomes unhidden in the joints) and arthritis ensues.

5 If Ying is taxed by heat, the Jing will step in and use its cold to hold the pathogen. When latency is lost from the Jing, heat along with the pathology is released, causing the Triple Heater pulse to float as it tries to clear the Jing of pathology. The pathogen then has access to the organs. Therefore the body will try at all costs to find an alternative reservoir of latency.

6 The Luo Channels can empty into the Yuan-Source level if they overflow with pathology and fail to find a neighboring Luo to occupy.

7 The Luos can empty into their related Primary Channel or a neighboring Luo.

8 Pathology in the Luos can find its way to the Eight Extra Channels. The last Yang Luo (the Gallbladder Luo) can empty its pathology to ST-42 which connects to Chong Mai, and the last Yin Luo (the Liver Luo) can empty into the Ren Mai at the end of its trajectory, CV-2, giving entry to the Constitution.

9 The Constitution can pass the pathology to its main reservoir, Dai Mai. When Dai Mai fills, it should drain, but if it cannot, it uses the Kidney Divergent Channel to extend its field of latency.

10 Once in a Divergent Channel, the pathogen can then move through the Divergent Channel sequence until it reaches the last confluence, the Large Intestine and Lung Divergent Channels.

11 At the end of the Divergent Channel sequence, the pathogen can enter the Primary Channels at ST-12, but the body will try to push the pathology to the Da Bao at GB-22 which is another point on the Lung Divergent Channel trajectory. GB-22 is also the Great Luo of the Spleen and the pathogen can find latency in the Luo arena there, also.

12 When The Great Luo of the Spleen fills, the pathology can spill down via either the GB Primary Channel or Bao Mai to Dai Mai, a major holding site.

13 At the end of the Divergent Channel sequence, the pathogen can go to Du Mai at GB-8.

14 When the capacity to hold the pathogen in latency is exhausted, the pathogen moves to the organs and the disease becomes life-threatening.

The Achievement of Latency of a Pathogenic Factor

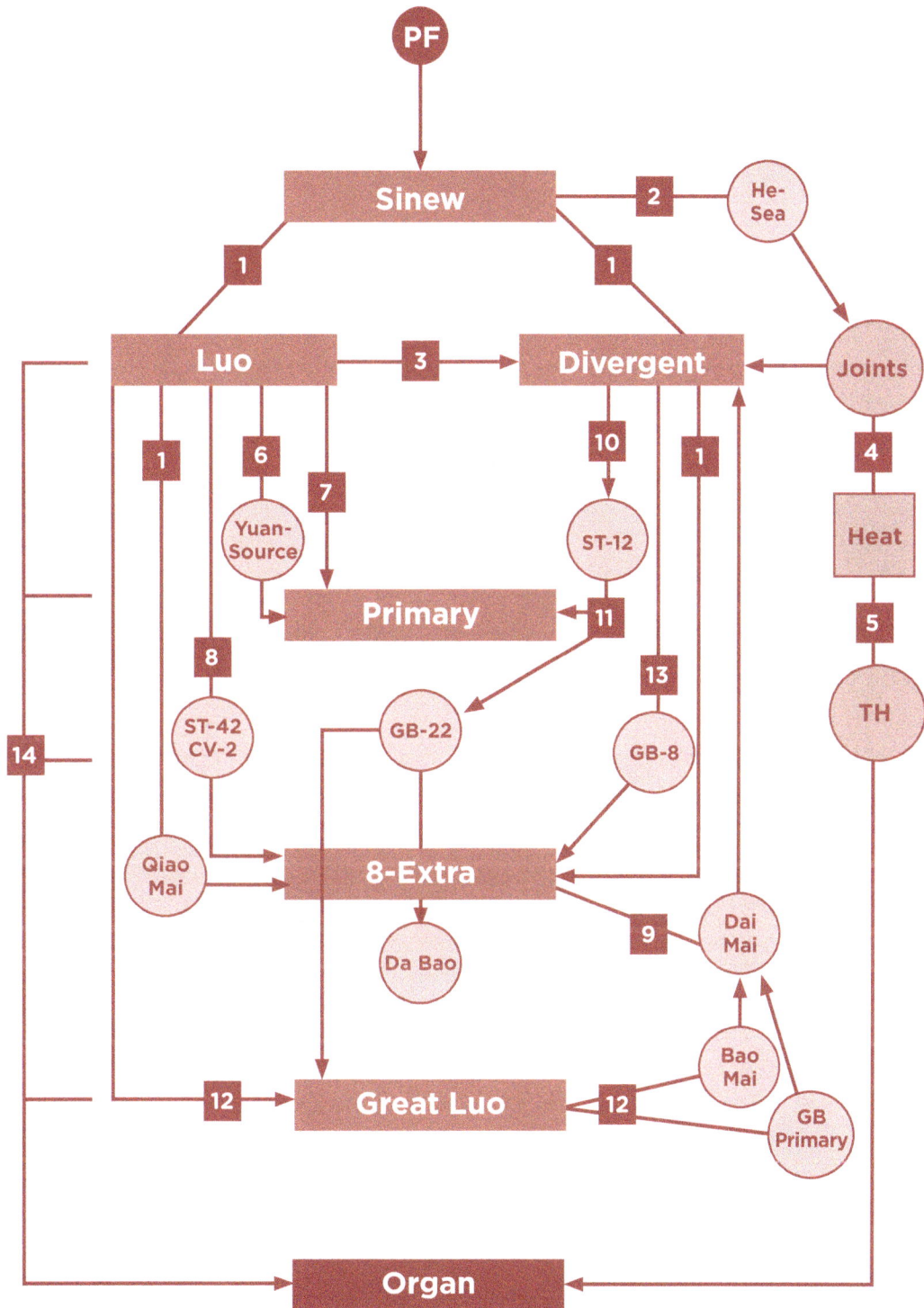

The human body recognizes that the disease of an internal organ is the most serious of all illnesses. Using very sophisticated strategies (described by the Complement Channels), the body shifts a pathogen out of the Primary Channels to ensure the safety of the organs or, in the case of the Sinew Channels, prevents penetration of the Primary Channels altogether. In the presence of a potentially life-threatening disease the Complement Channels move the illness away from the Zang Fu, and can create a different disease so that the viscera are preserved; they shift an acute condition into latency or they create a "slower" disease. The Complement Channels are present literally to preserve humanity.

The Organization and Terrain of the Complement Channels

Channel	Qi Levels		
	Wei	Ying	Yuan
12 Sinew Channels	✓		
6 Cutaneous regions	✓		
12 Primary Channels	✓	✓	
16 Luo Channels		✓	
12 Divergent Channels	✓		✓
8 Extraordinary Channels			✓
2 bisecting or cross-sectioning connections		✓	✓

The Terrain of the Channels

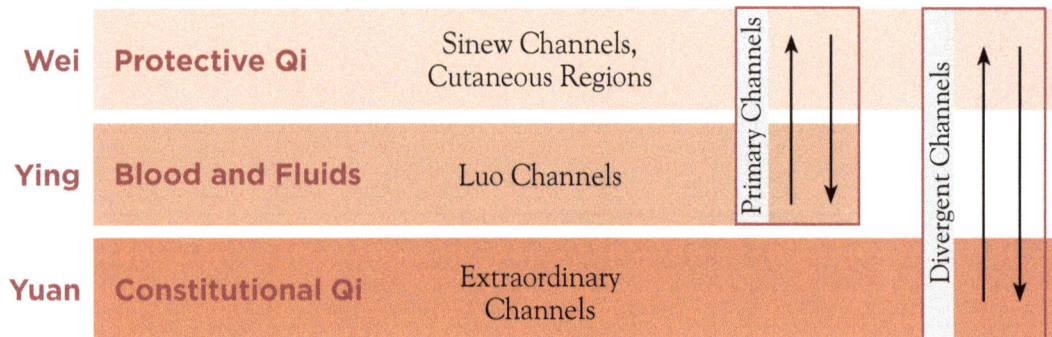

			Primary Channels	Divergent Channels
Wei	**Protective Qi**	Sinew Channels, Cutaneous Regions		
Ying	**Blood and Fluids**	Luo Channels		
Yuan	**Constitutional Qi**	Extraordinary Channels		

The Sinew Channels

Bladder Sinew Channel

Jing Well point: BL-67
Confluent point: SI-18

SINEW

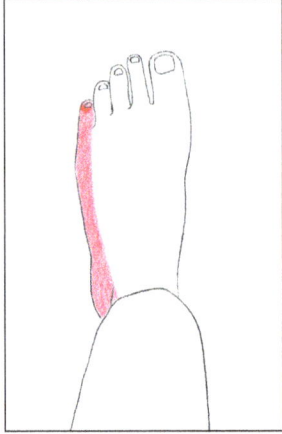

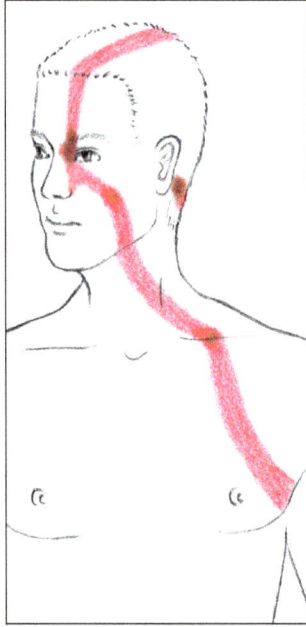

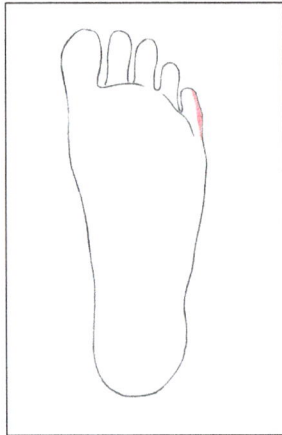

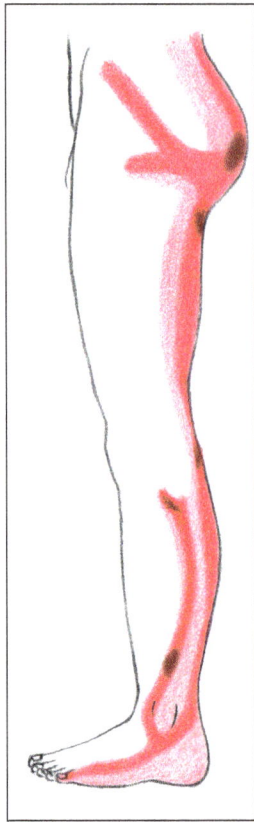

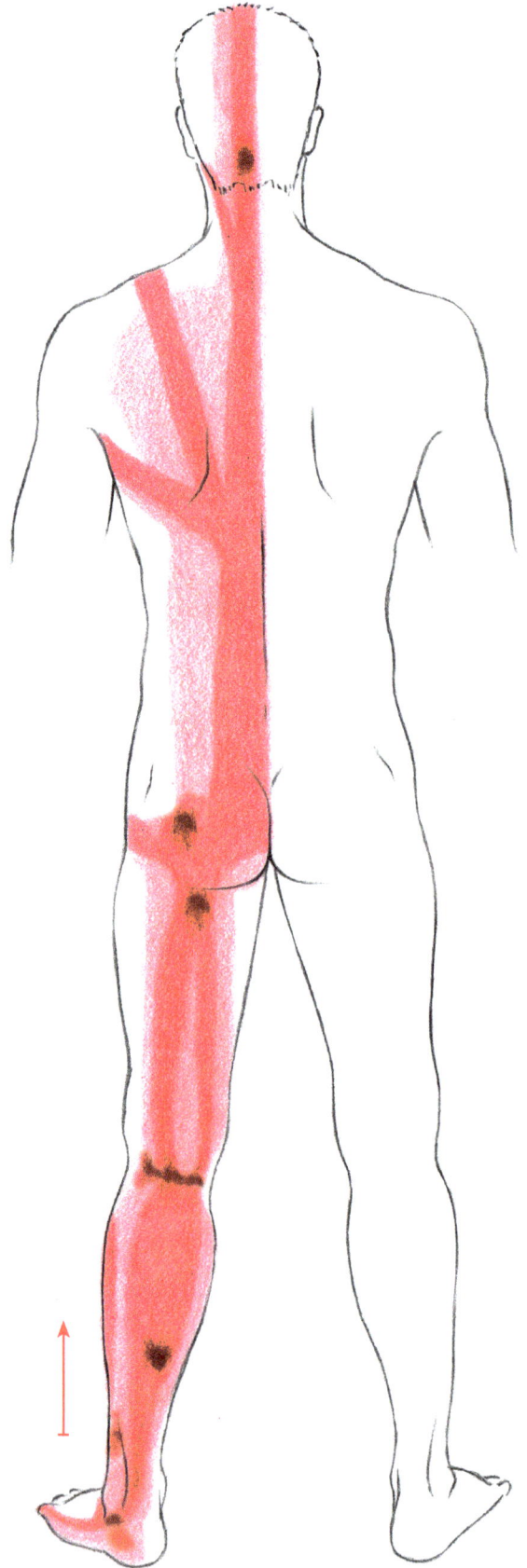

Jing Well point: GB-44

Confluent point: SI-18

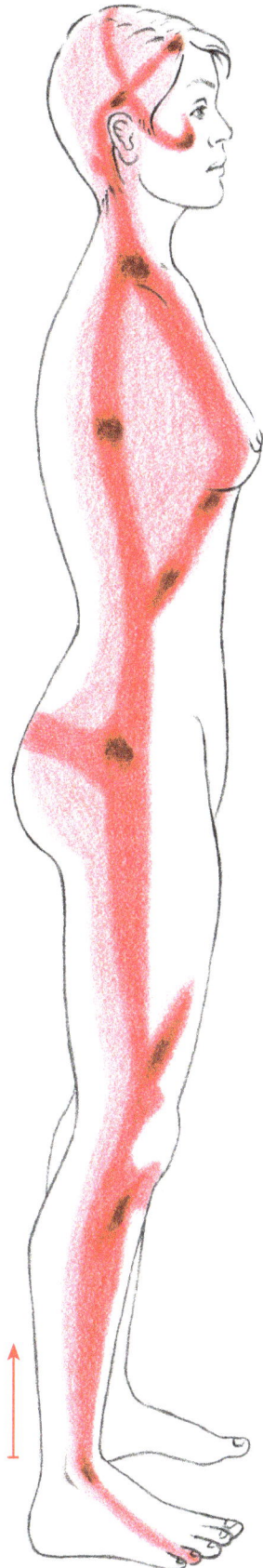

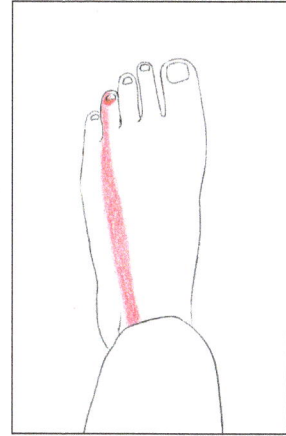

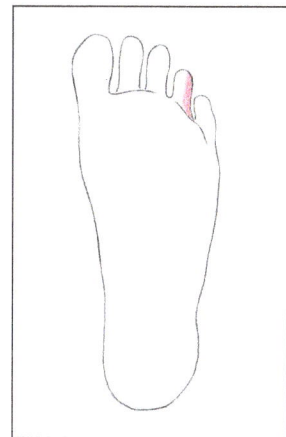

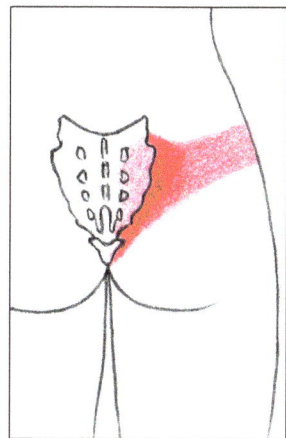

Stomach Sinew Channel

Jing Well point: ST-45
Confluent point: SI-18

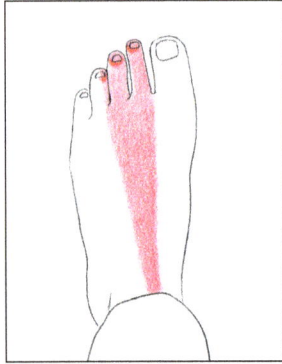

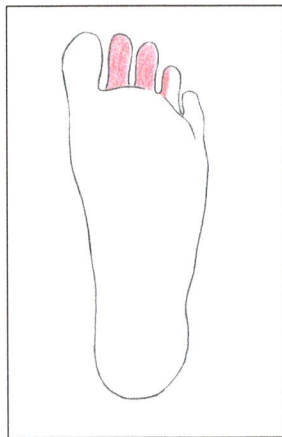

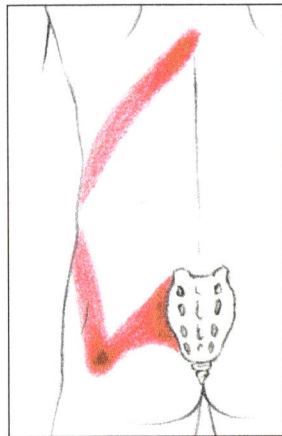

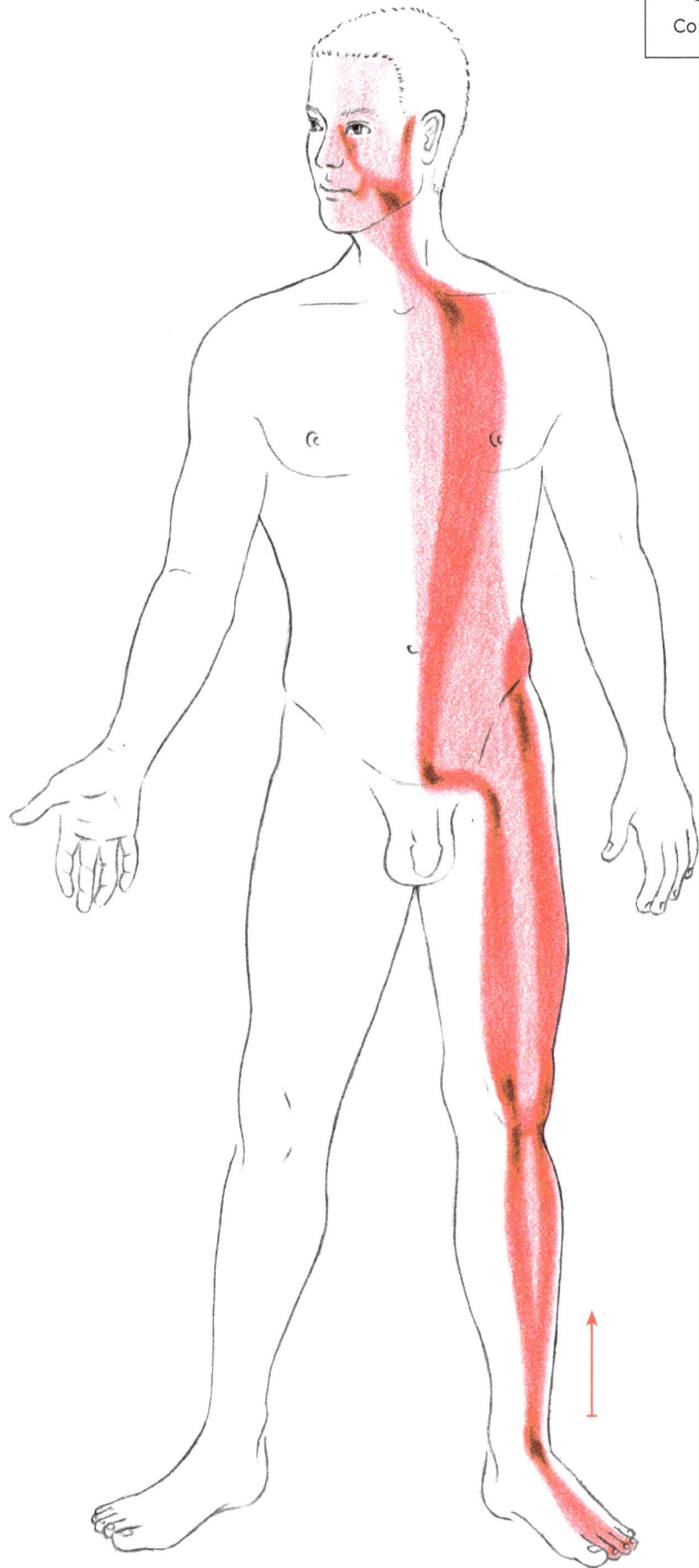

Jing Well point: SI-1

Confluent point: ST-8

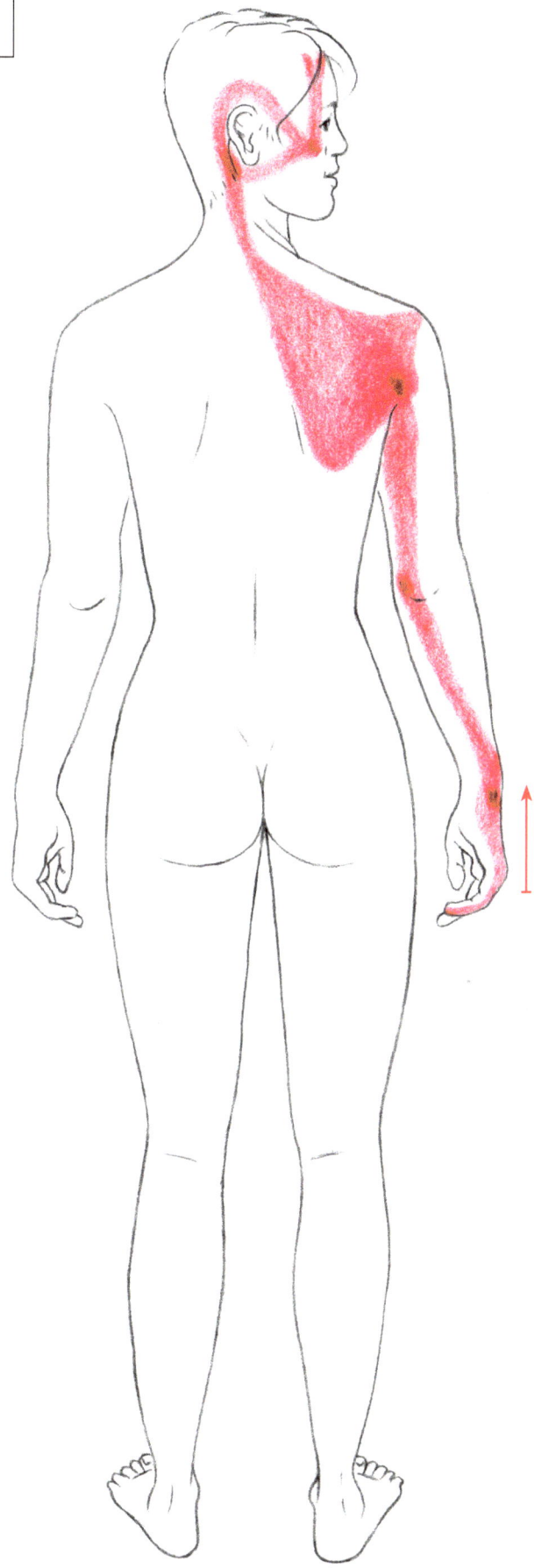

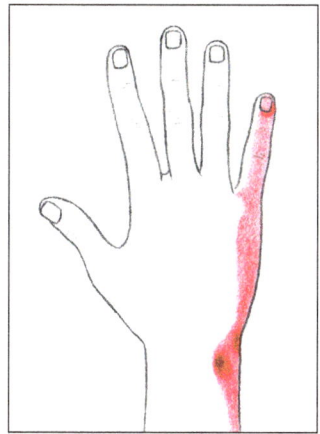

Triple Heater Sinew Channel

Jing Well point: TH-1

Confluent point: ST-8

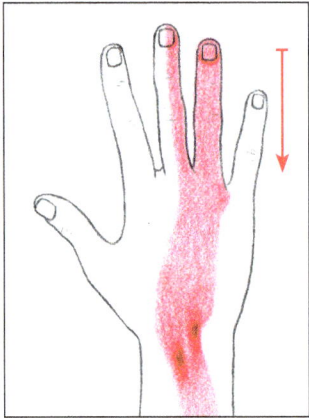

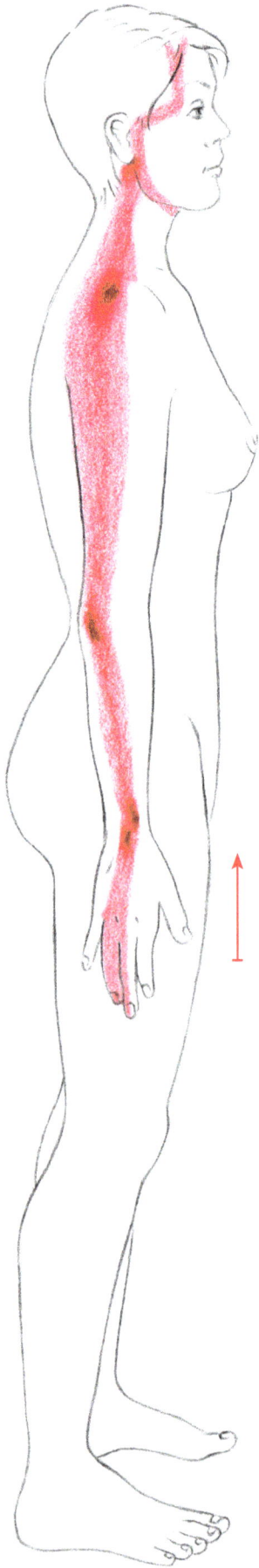

Large Intestine Sinew Channel

Jing Well point: LI-1

Confluent point: ST-8

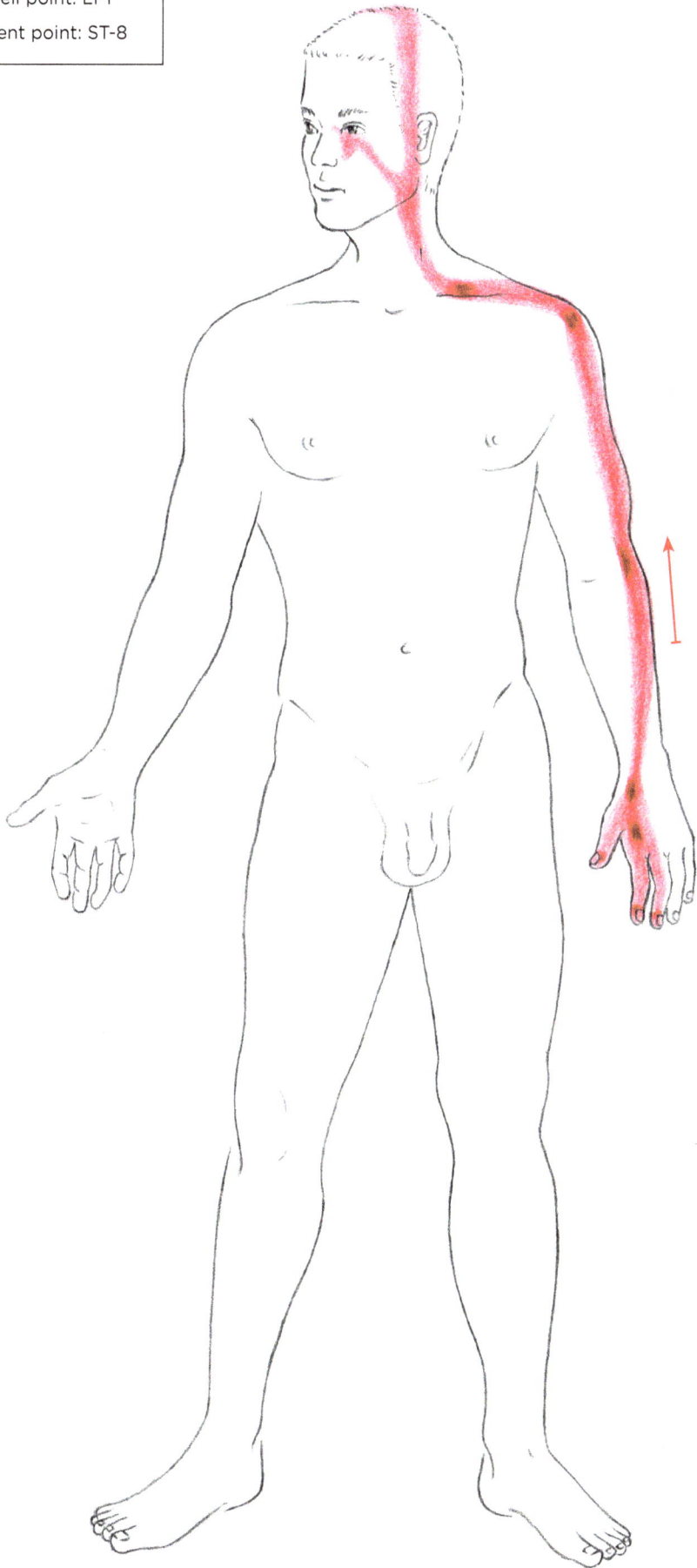

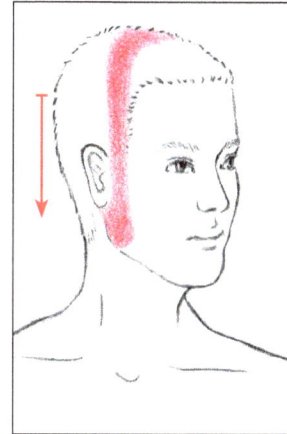

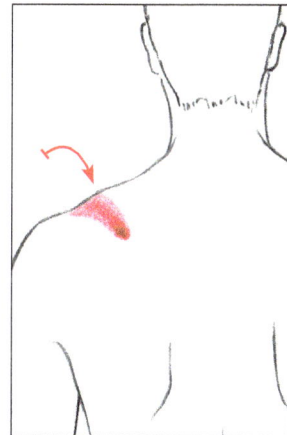

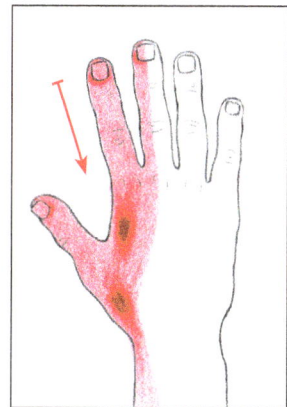

7

Spleen Sinew Channel

Jing Well point: SP-1

Confluent point: CV-3

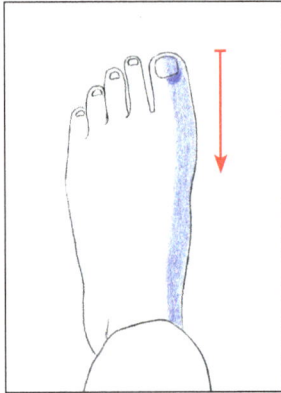

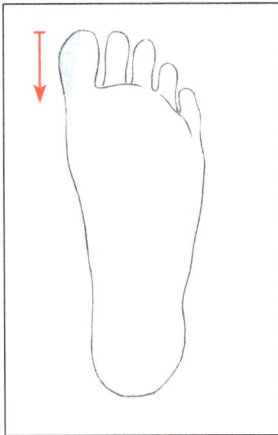

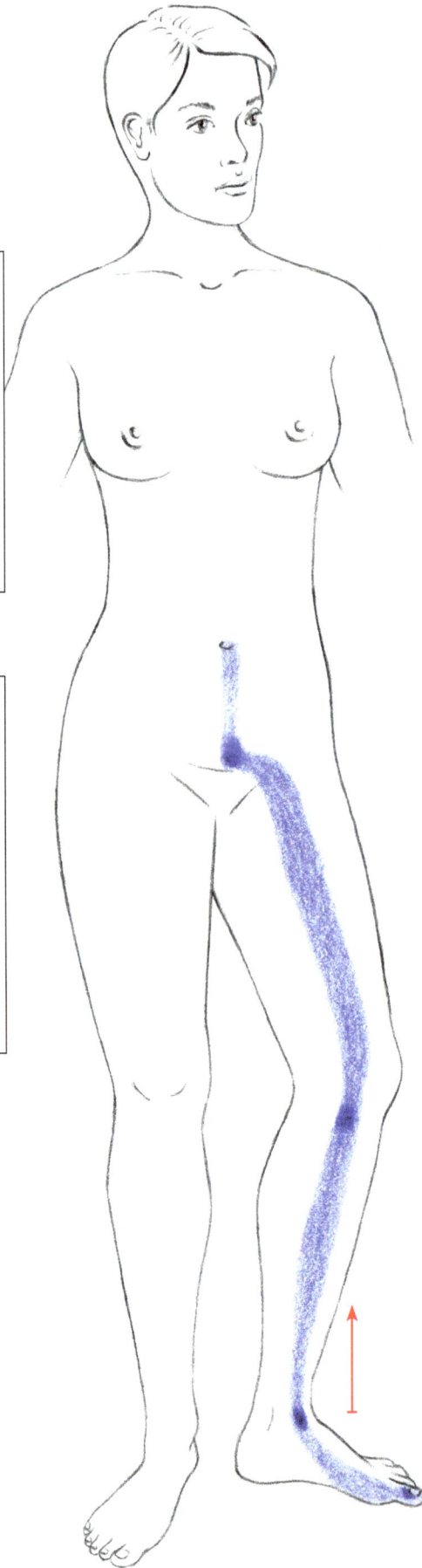

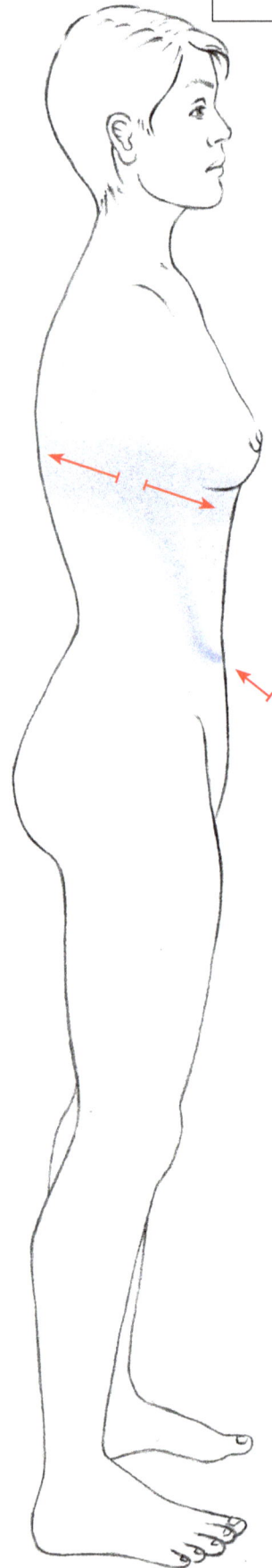

Jing Well point: LU-11

Confluent point: GB-22

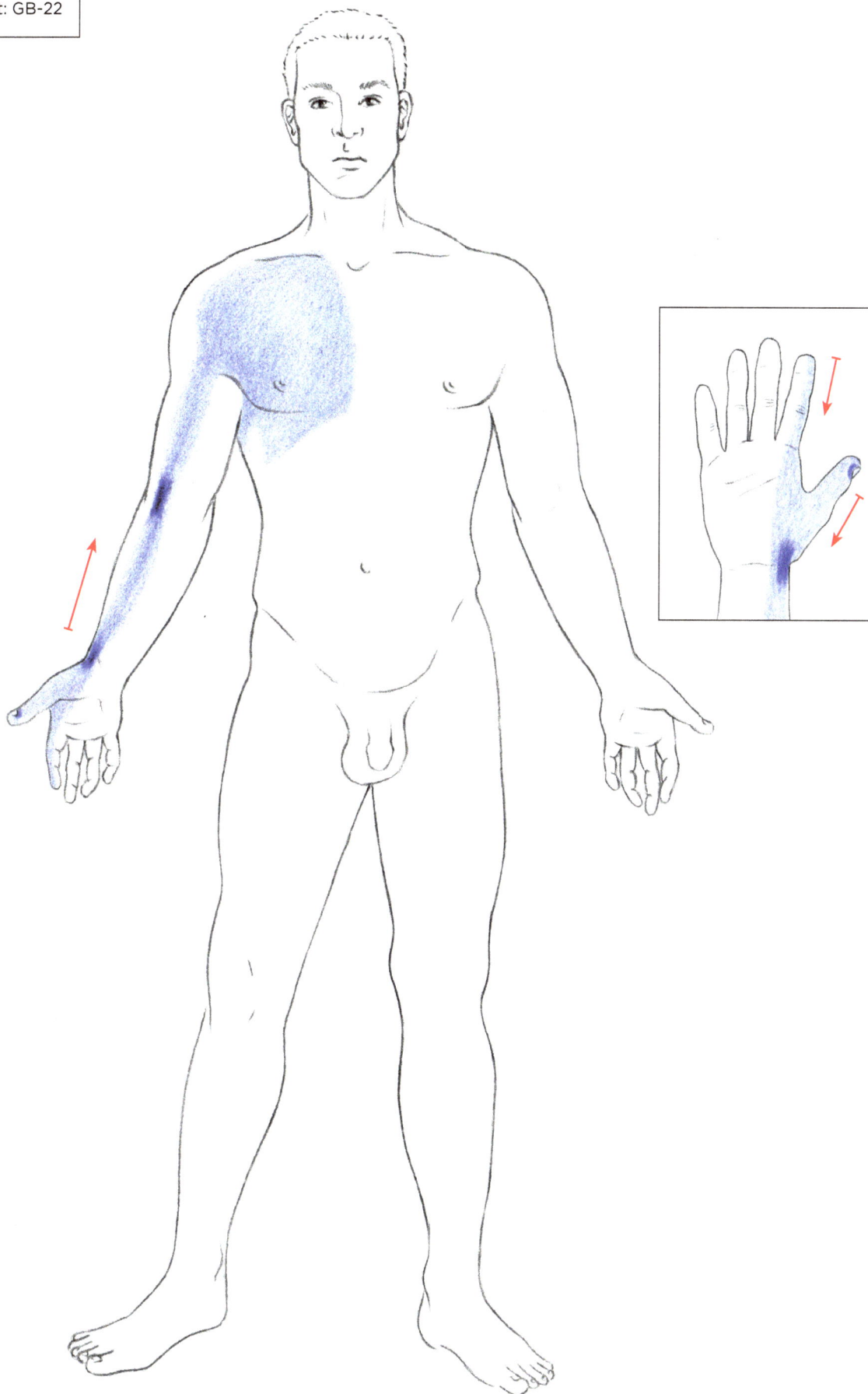

Kidney Sinew Channel

Jing Well point: KI-1
Confluent point: CV-3

SINEW

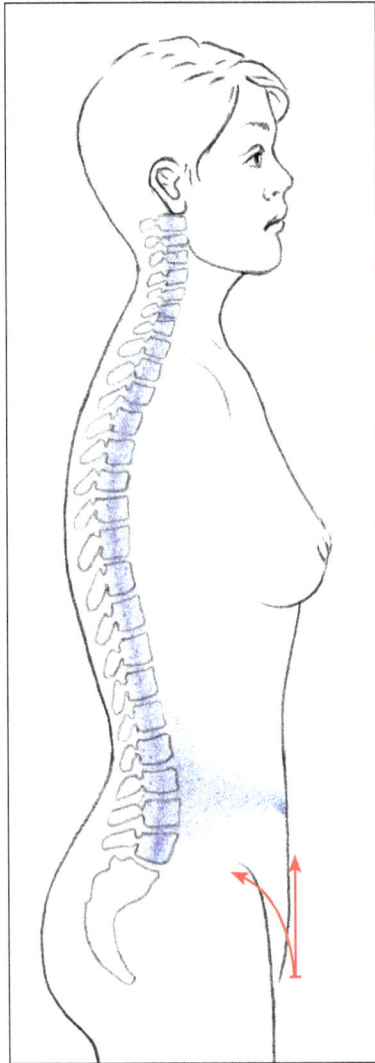

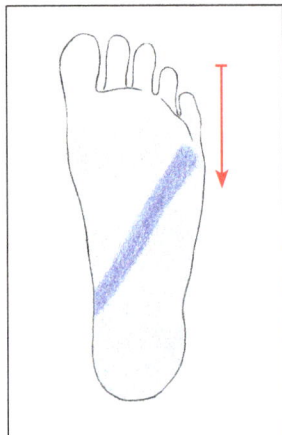

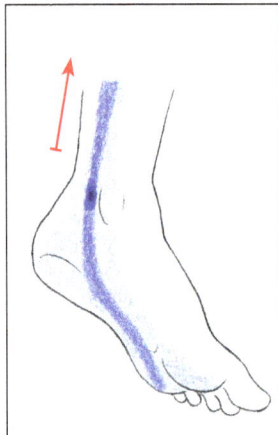

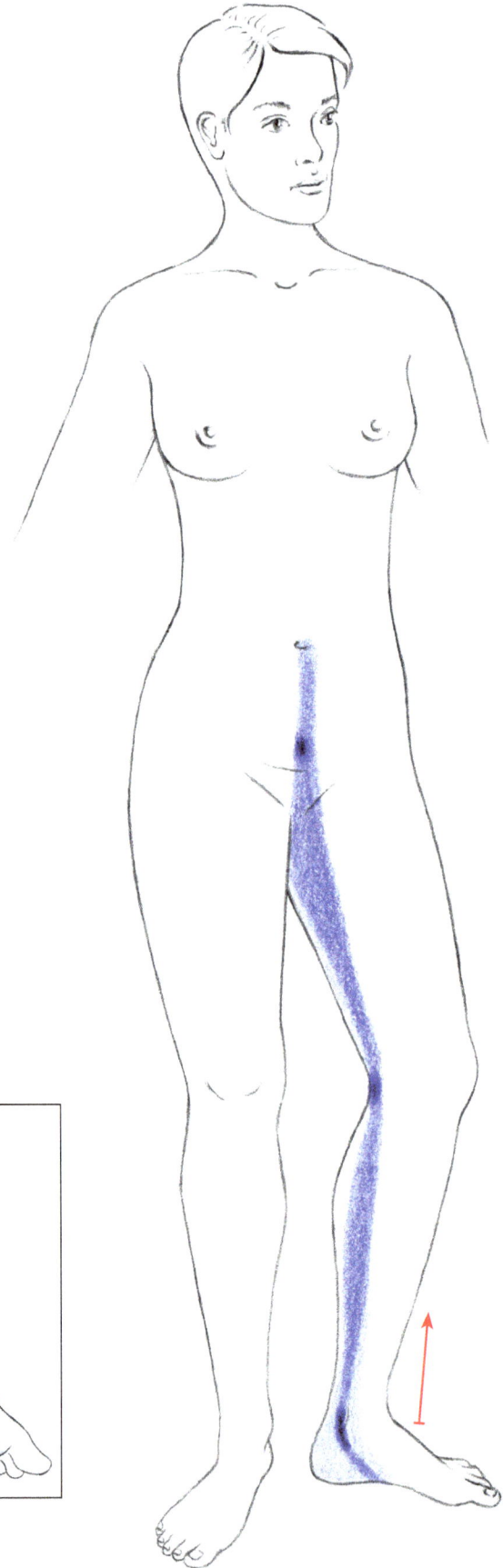

Jing Well point: HT-9

Confluent point: GB-22

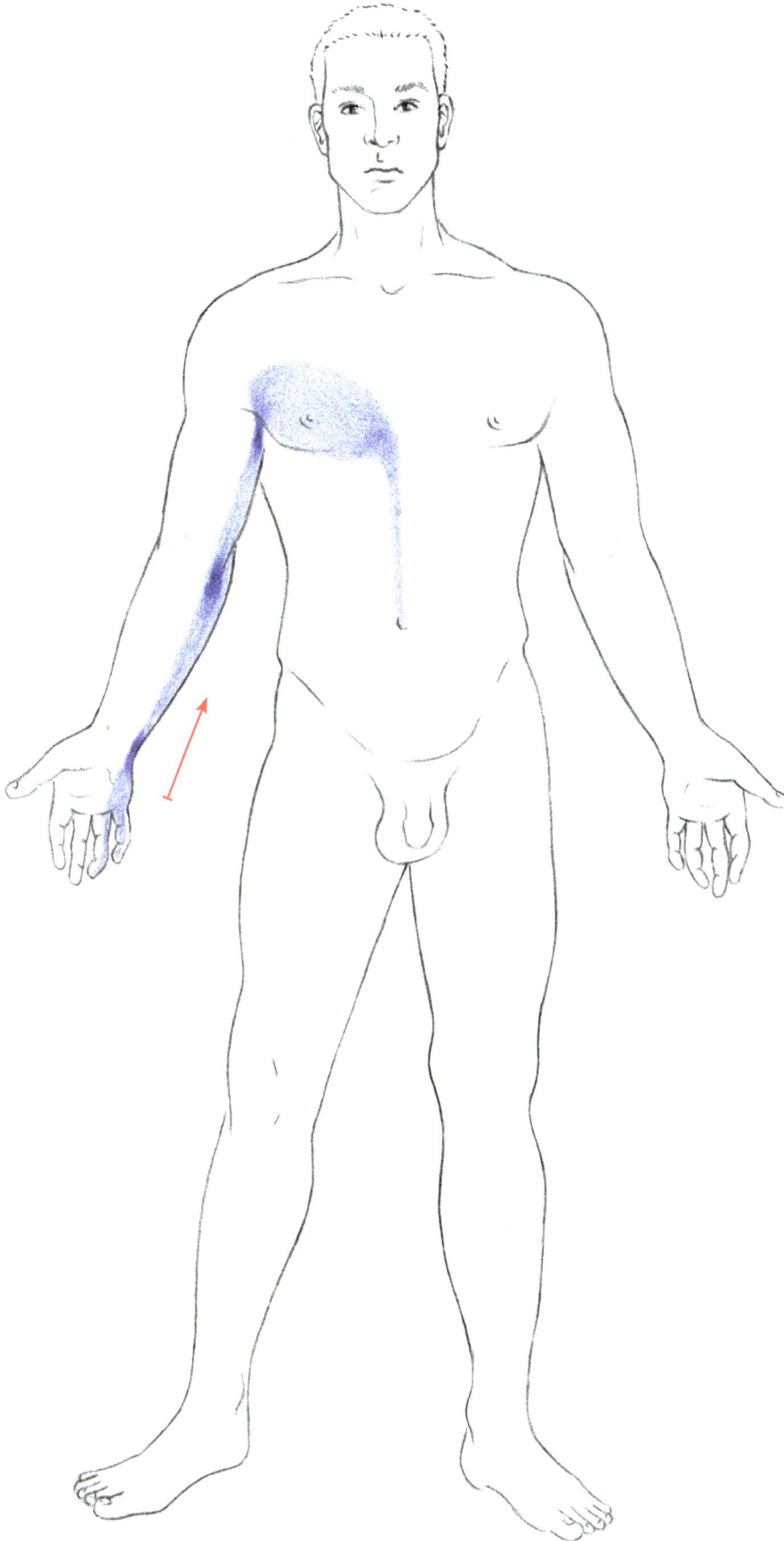

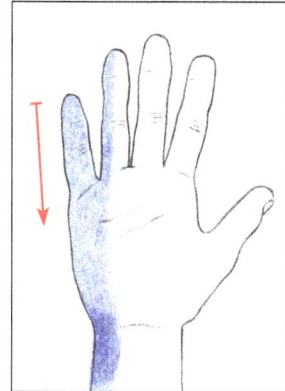

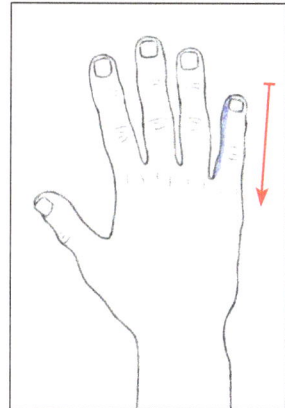

Liver Sinew Channel

Jing Well point: LR-1
Confluent point: CV-3

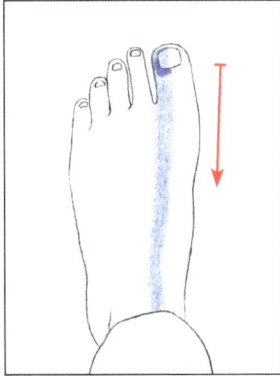

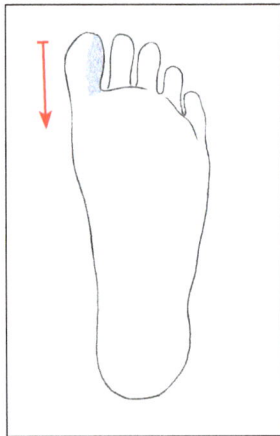

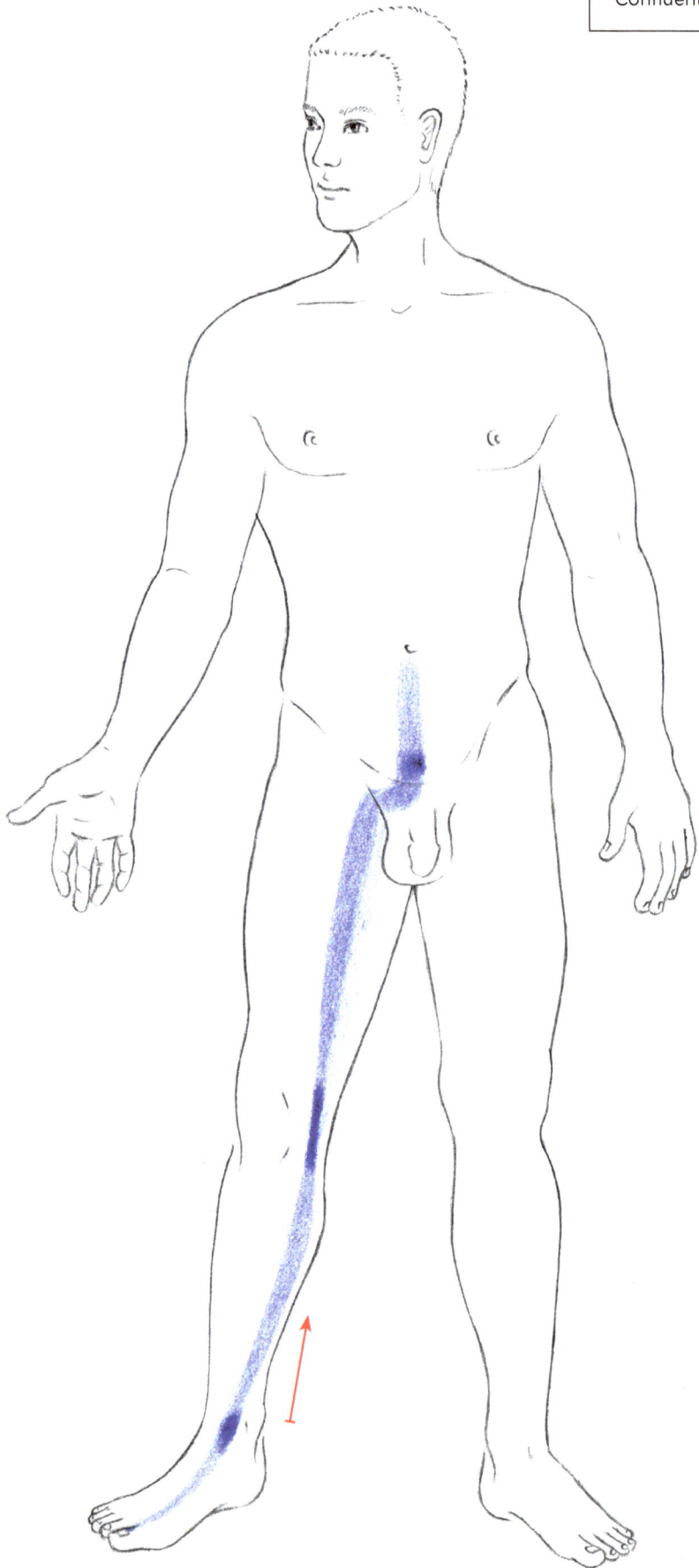

12

Jing Well point: PC-9

Confluent point: GB-22

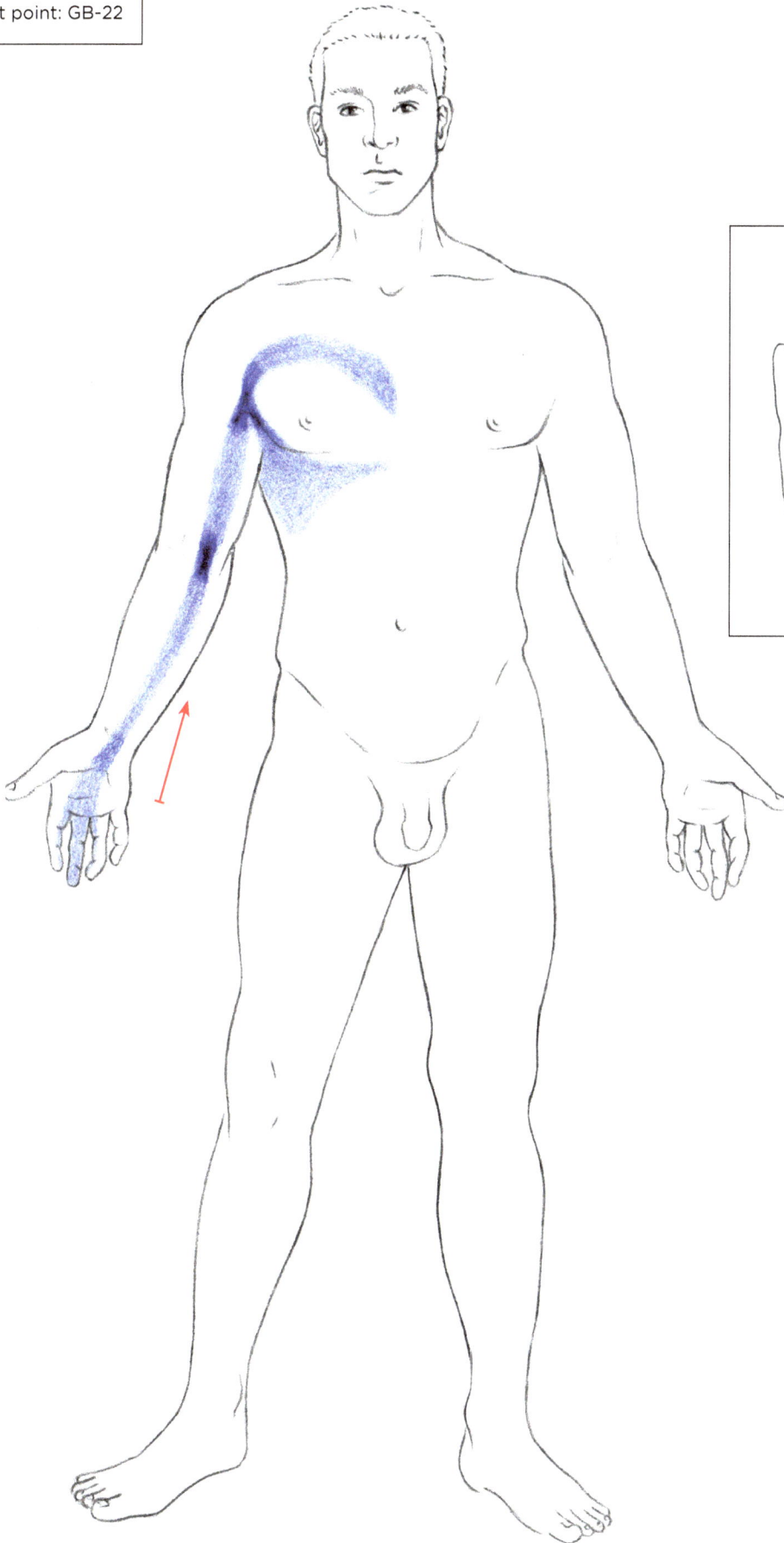

The Luo Channels

* It should be noted that there are no points along the Luo Channel trajectories other than the Luo point itself. The Luos traverse areas, feathering out and dispersing along the way. Choose bleeding sites according to where you actually see Luo vessels.

Lung Luo Channel

Luo point, LU-7
Longitudinal Luo
Transverse First Segment
Transverse Second Segment

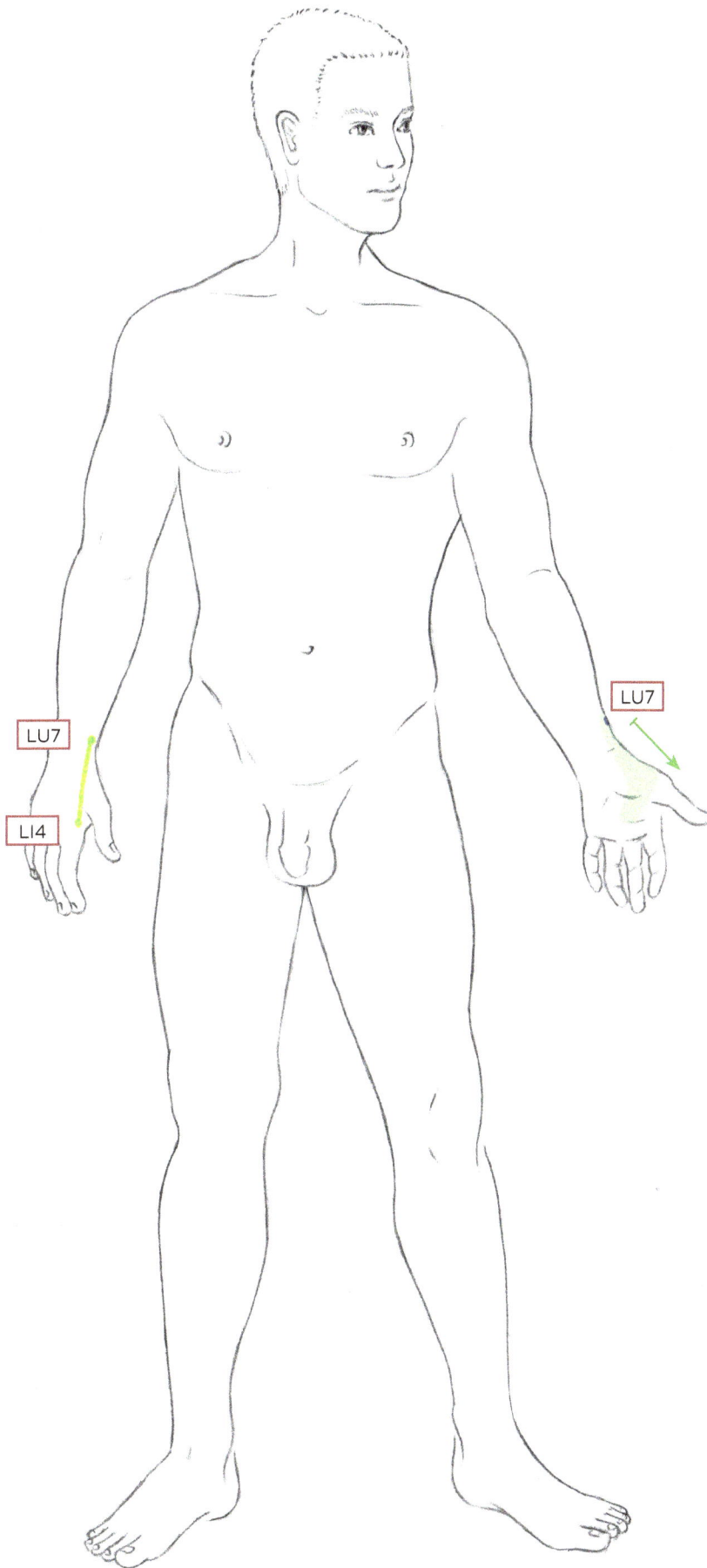

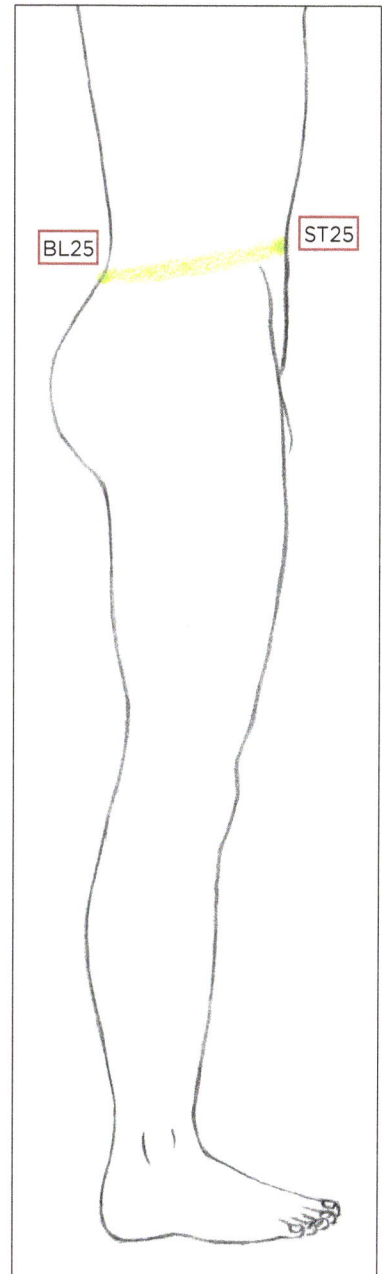

LU7

LU7

LI4

BL25

ST25

15

Large Intestine Luo Channel

Luo point, LI-6
Longitudinal Luo
Transverse First Segment
Transverse Second Segment

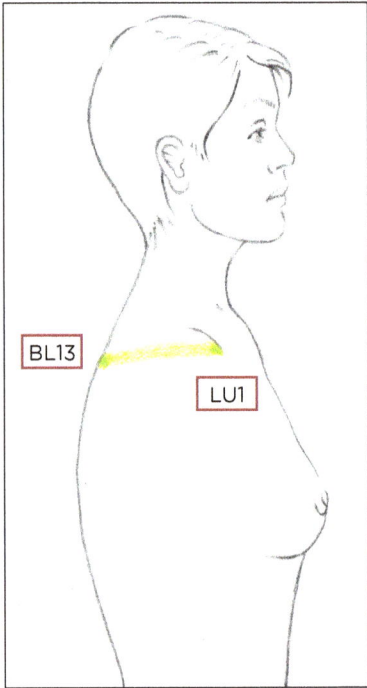

BL13

LU1

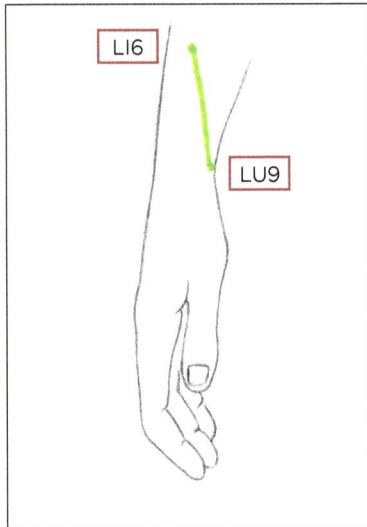

LI6

LU9

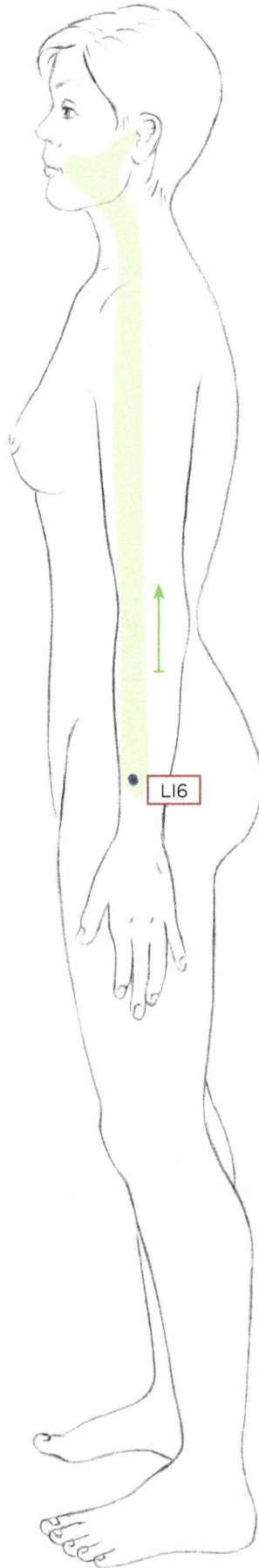

LI6

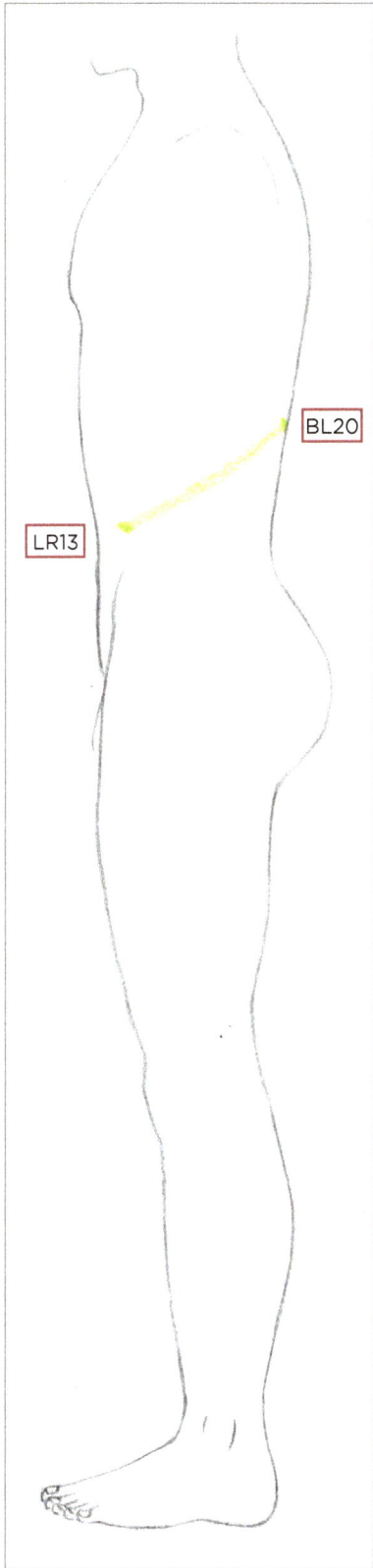

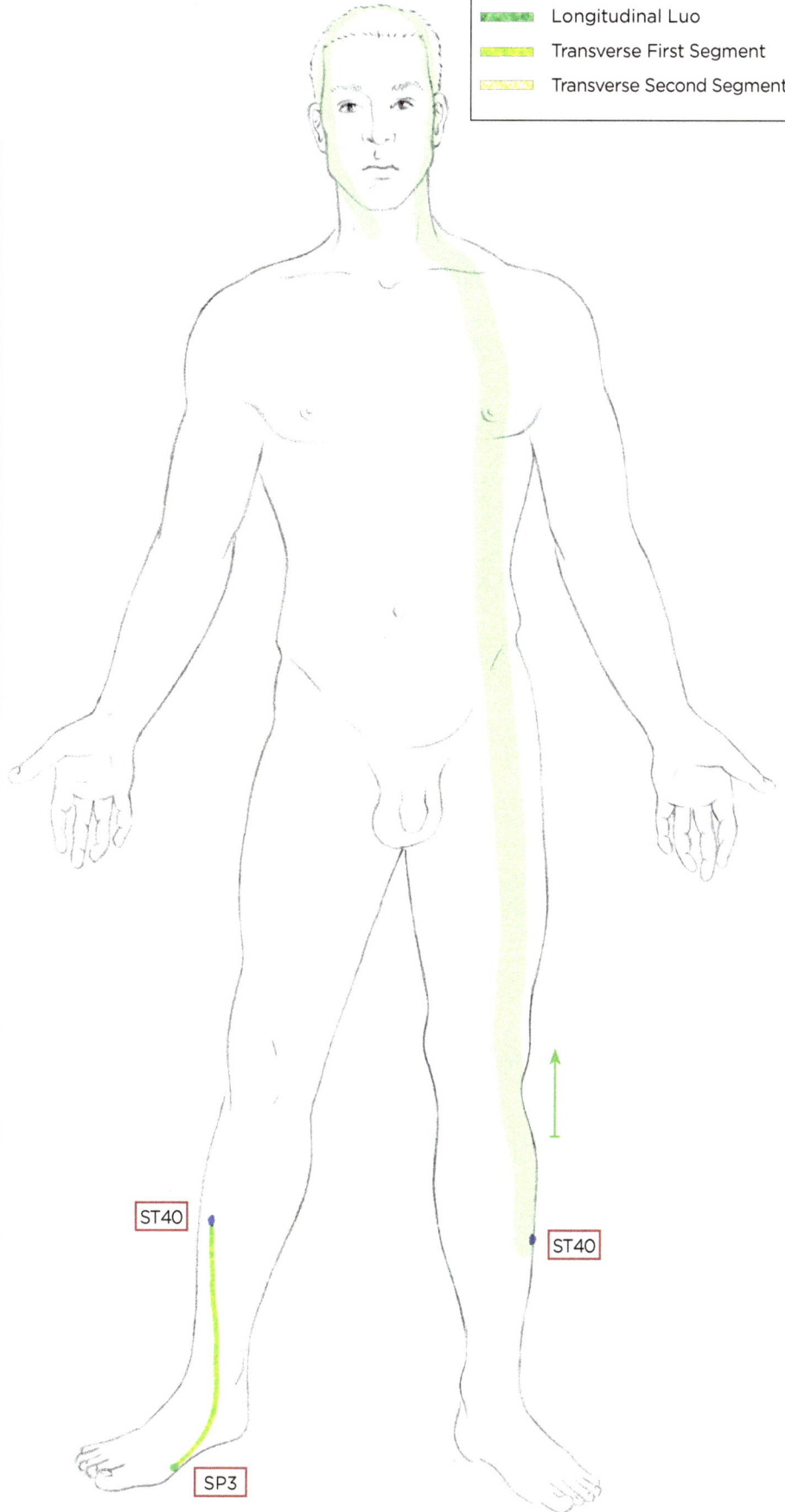

Luo point, ST-40
Longitudinal Luo
Transverse First Segment
Transverse Second Segment

LUO

BL20

LR13

ST40

ST40

SP3

17

Spleen Luo Channel

Luo point, SP-4
Longitudinal Luo
Transverse First Segment
Transverse Second Segment

LUO

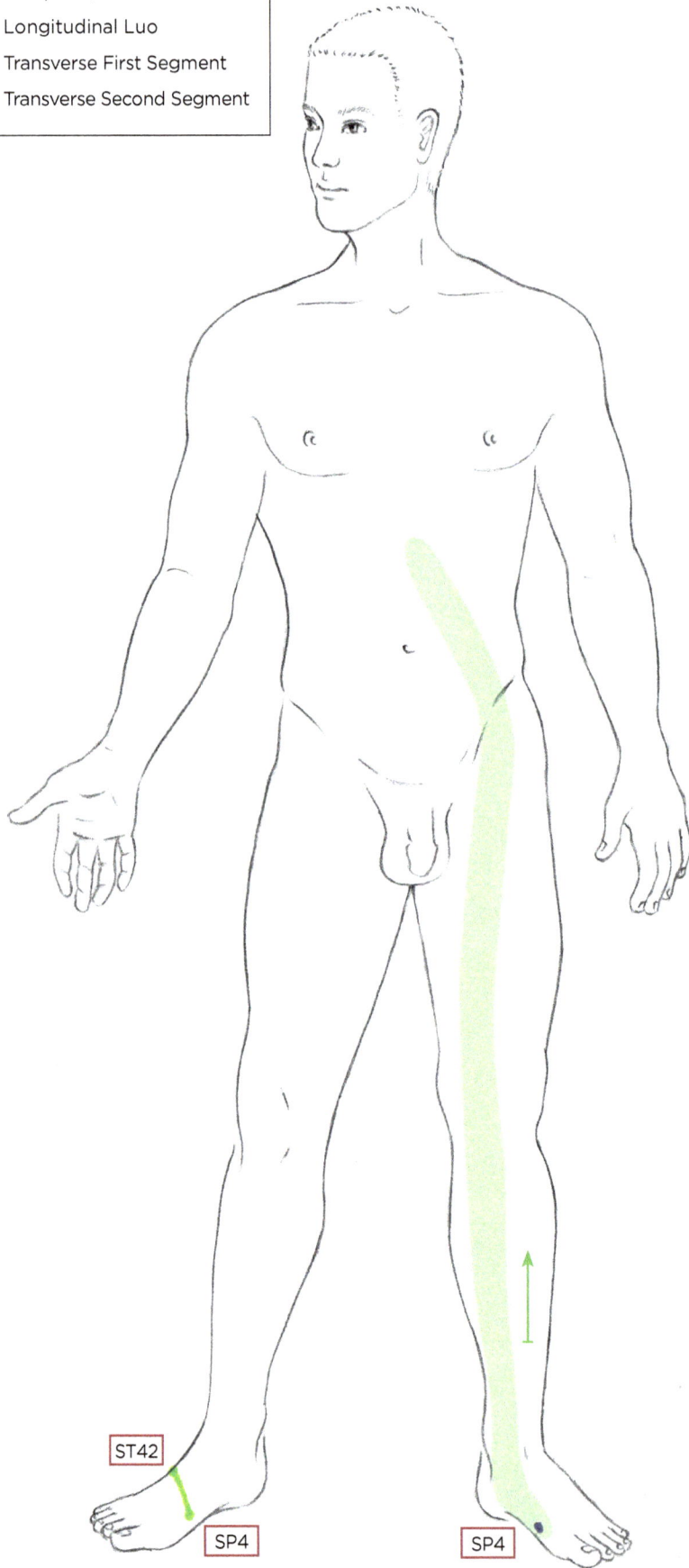

ST42

SP4

SP4

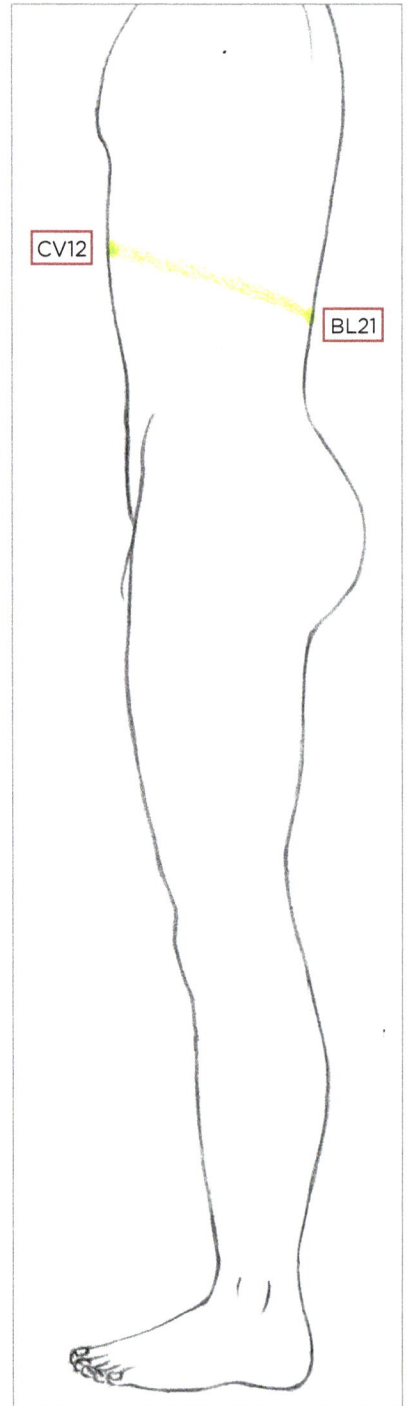

CV12

BL21

Luo point, HT-5
Longitudinal Luo
Transverse First Segment
Transverse Second Segment

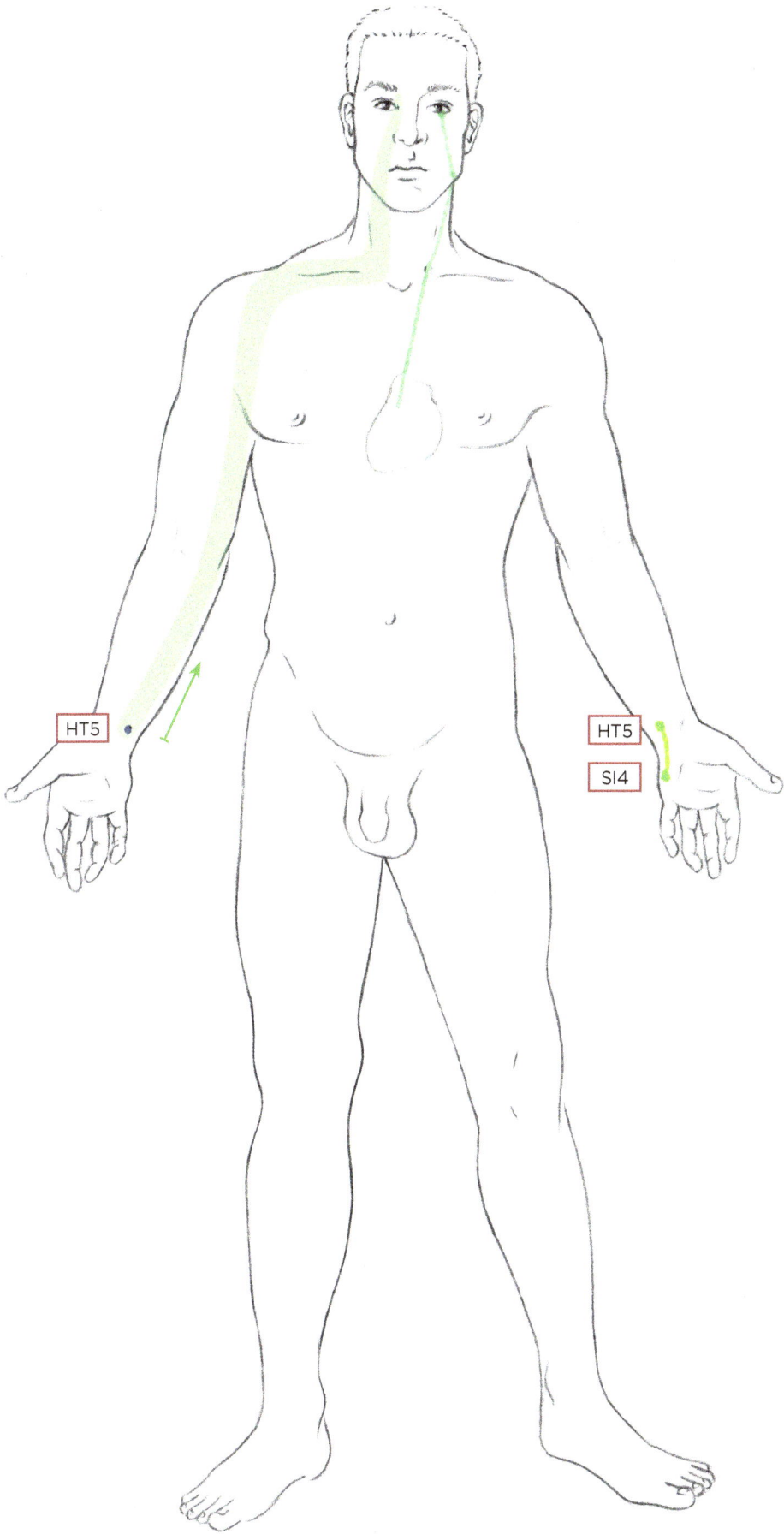

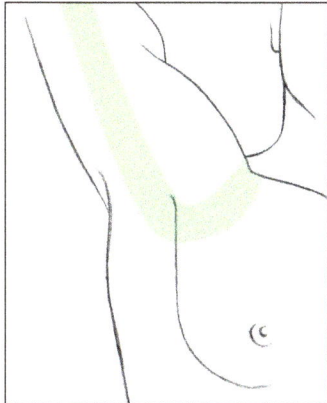

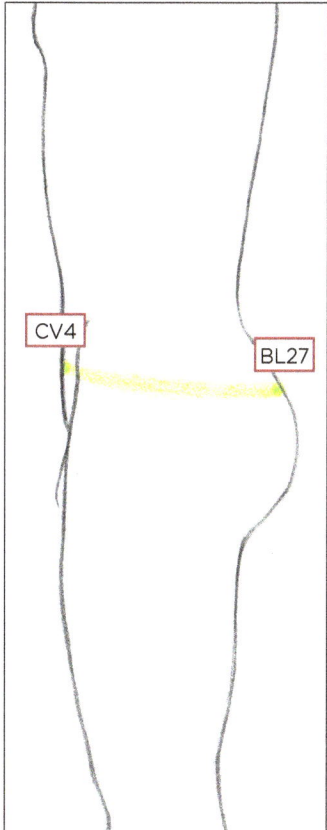

LUO

HT5

HT5

SI4

CV4

BL27

19

Small Intestine Luo Channel

Luo point, SI-7
Longitudinal Luo
Transverse First Segment
Transverse Second Segment

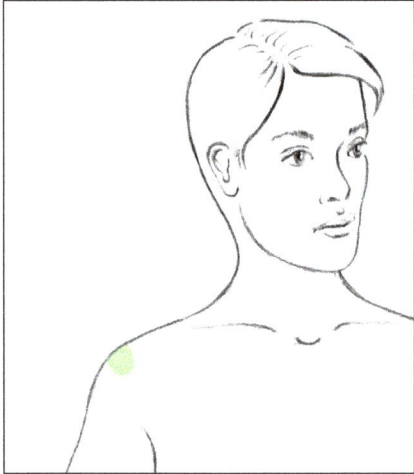

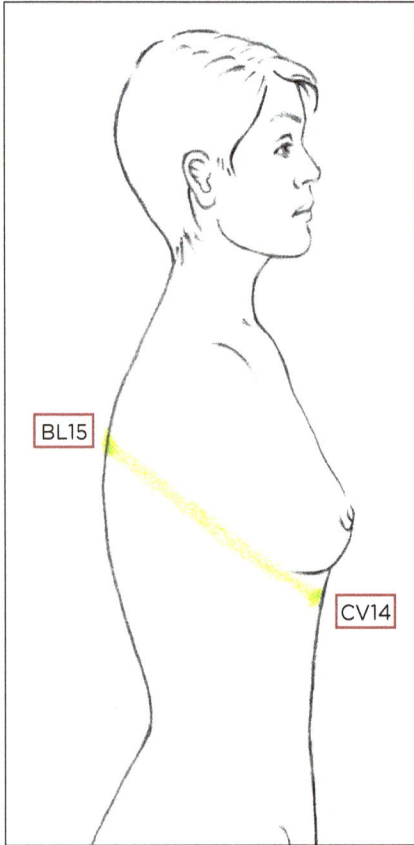

BL15

CV14

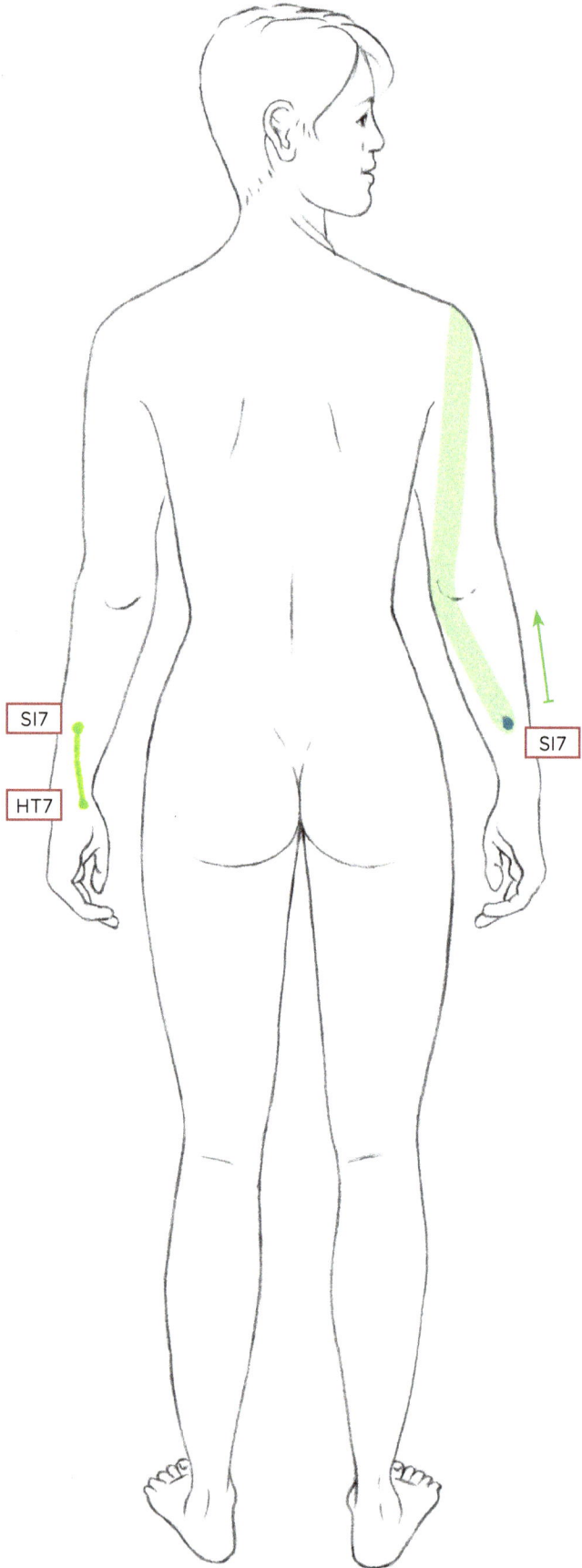

SI7

HT7

SI7

20

Bladder Luo Channel

Luo point, BL-58
Longitudinal Luo
Transverse First Segment
Transverse Second Segment

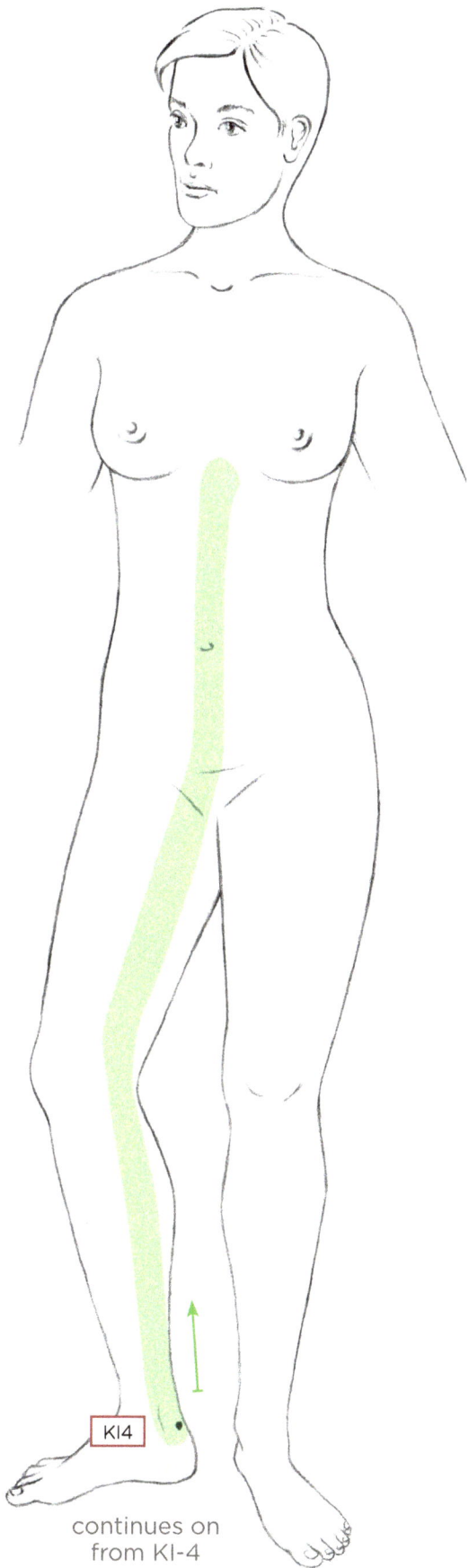

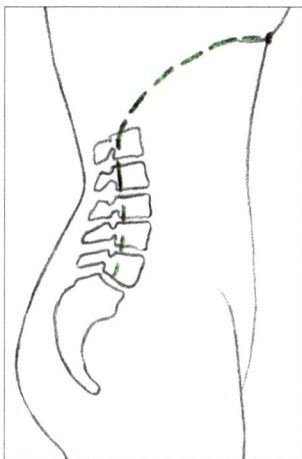

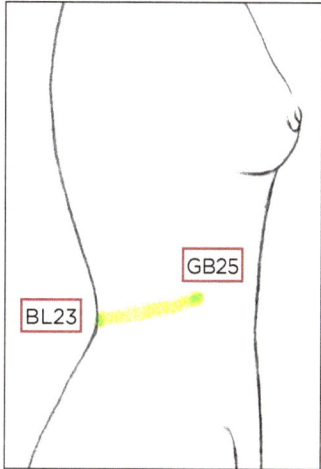

GB25

BL23

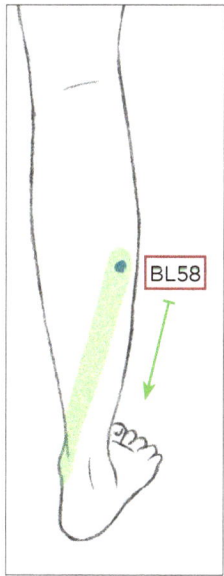

BL58

Begins here

KI4

continues on
from KI-4

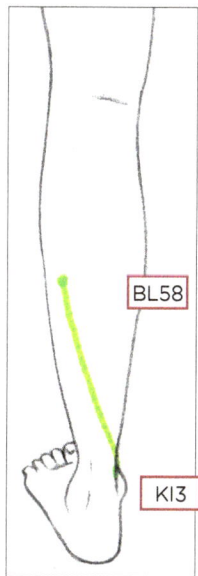

BL58

KI3

21

Kidney Luo Channel

Luo point, KI-4
Longitudinal Luo
Transverse First Segment
Transverse Second Segment

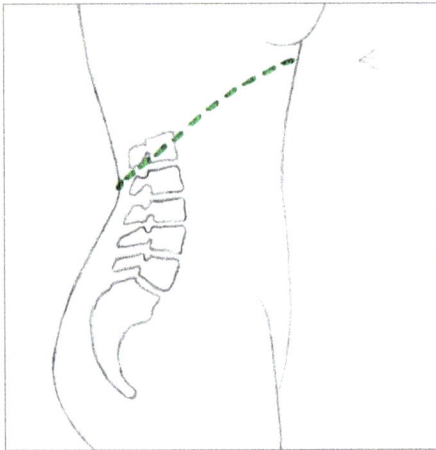

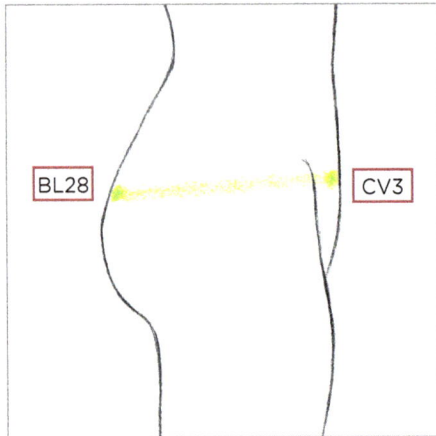

BL28   CV3

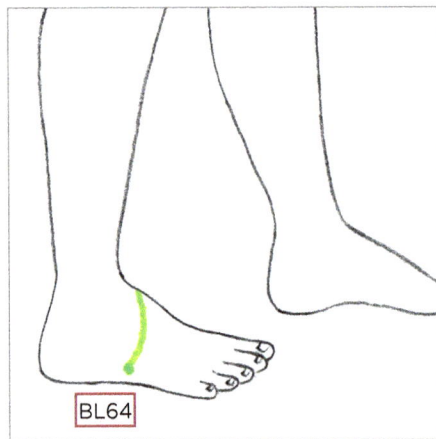

BL64

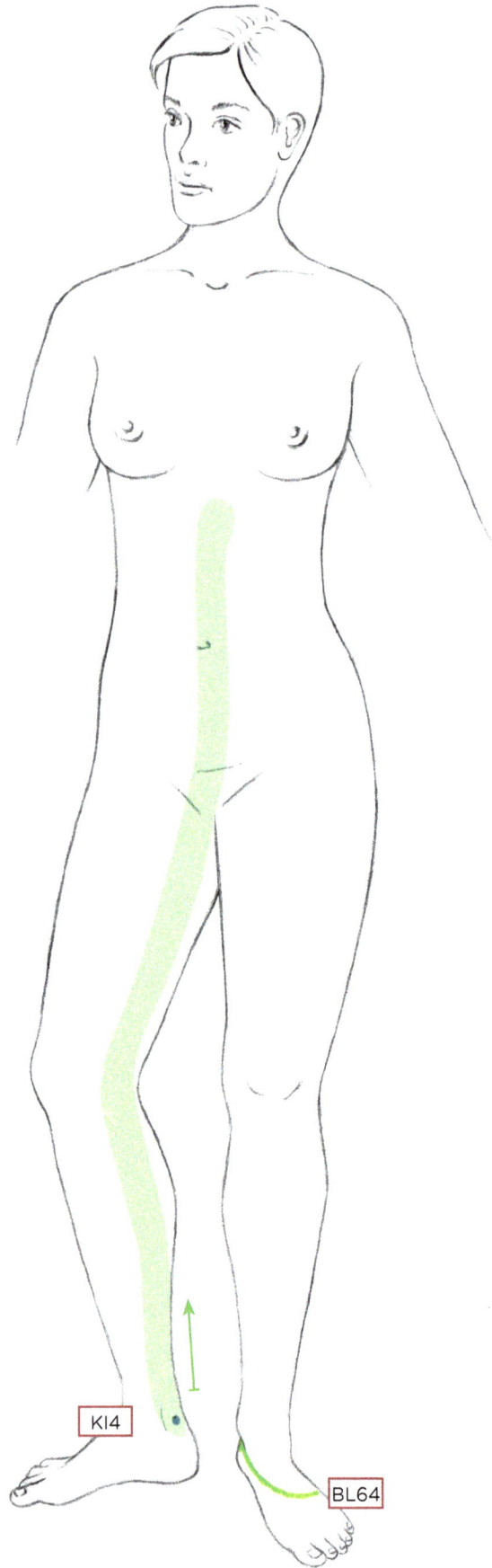

KI4   BL64

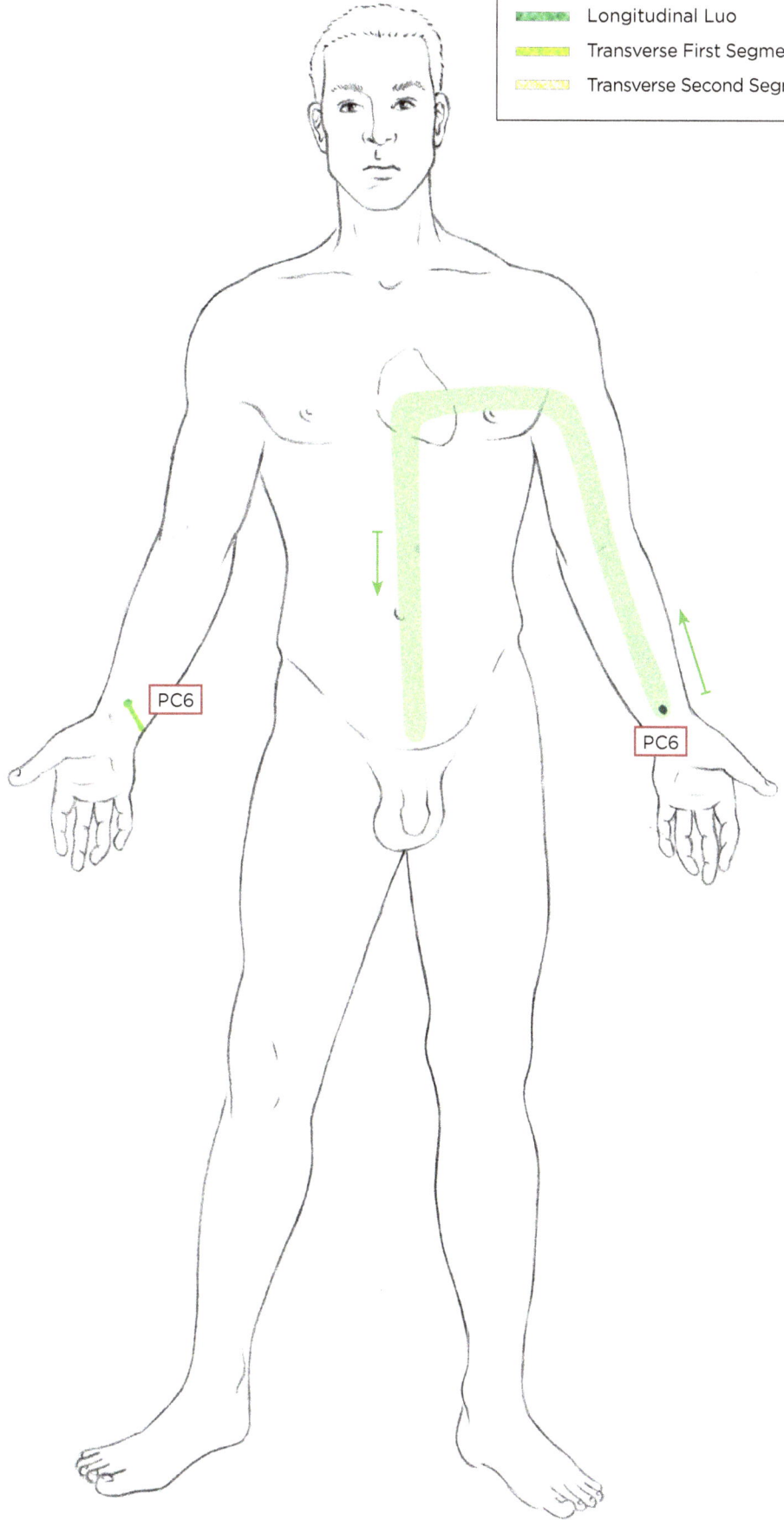

Pericardium Luo Channel

	Luo point, PC-6
	Longitudinal Luo
	Transverse First Segment
	Transverse Second Segment

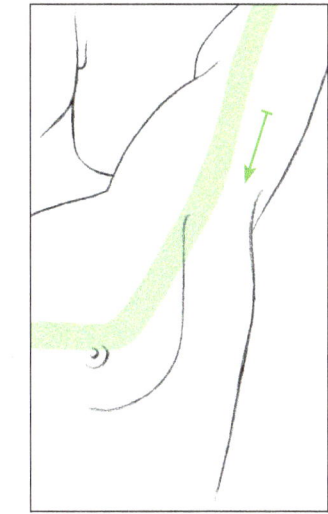

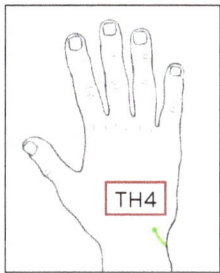

PC6

PC6

TH4

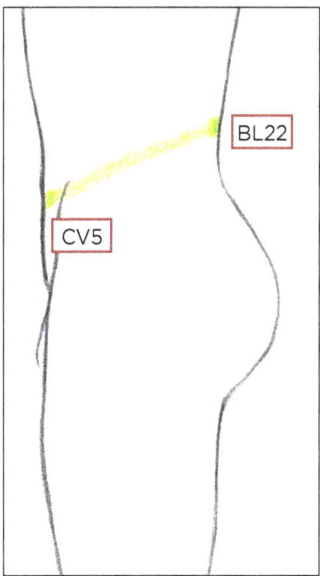

BL22

CV5

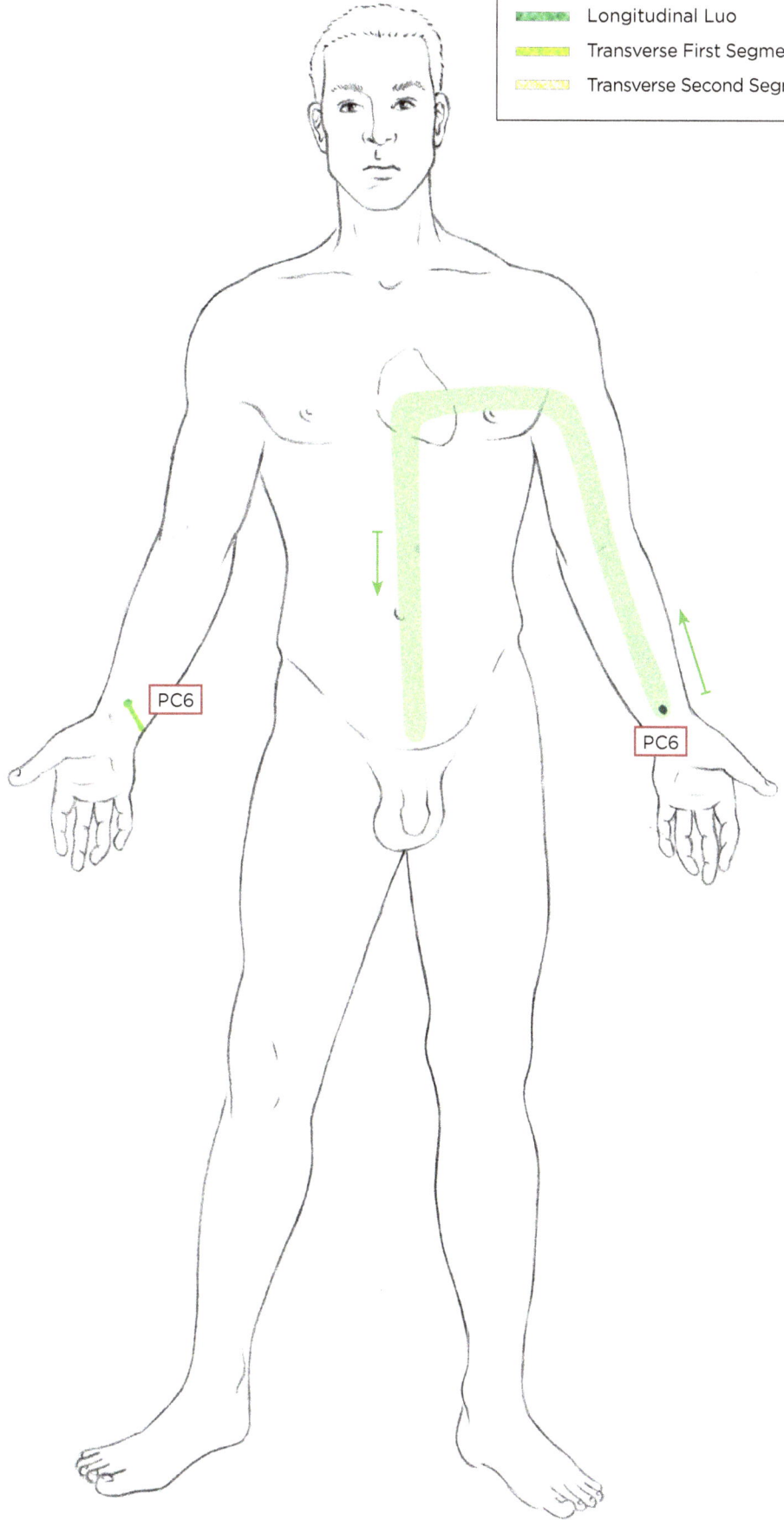

LUO

Triple Heater Luo Channel

●	Luo point, TH-5
▬	Longitudinal Luo
▬	Transverse First Segment
▬	Transverse Second Segment

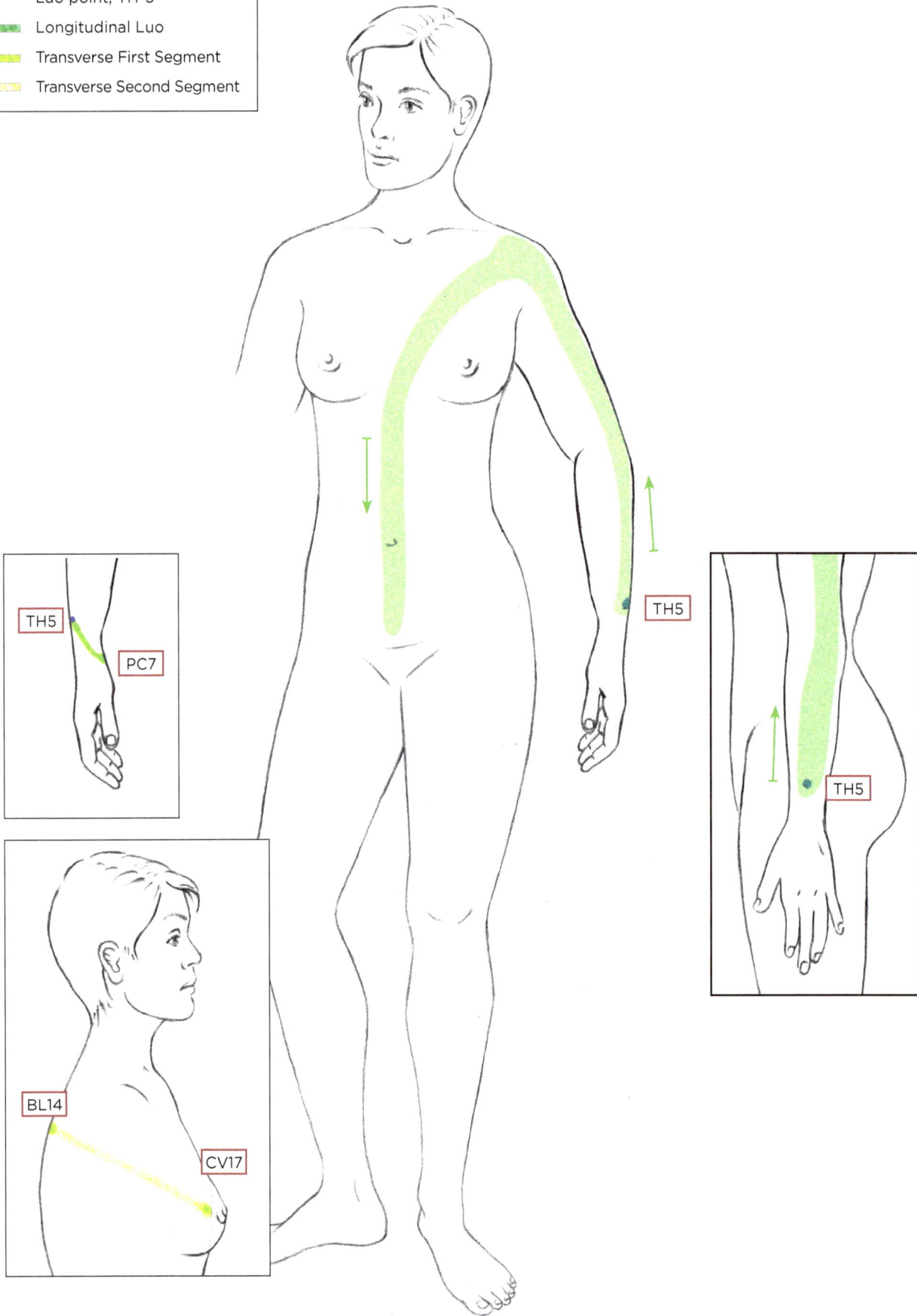

TH5

PC7

TH5

TH5

BL14

CV17

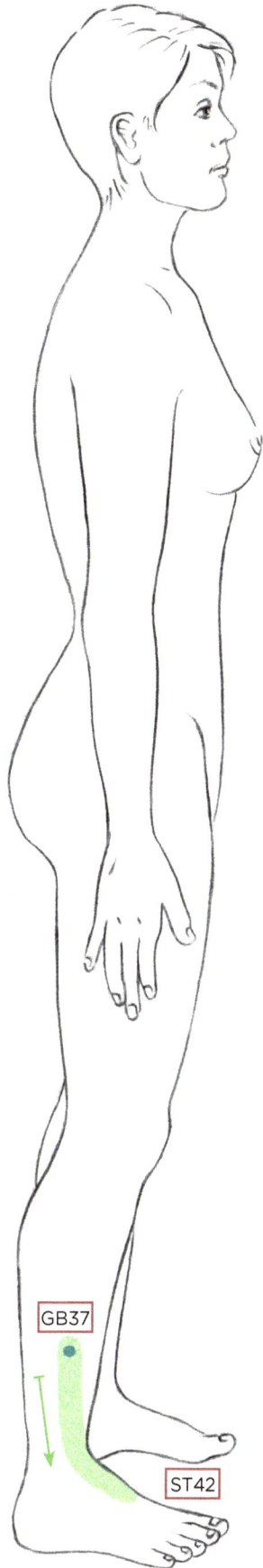

Gallbladder Luo Channel

	Luo point, GB-37
	Longitudinal Luo
	Transverse First Segment
	Transverse Second Segment

LUO

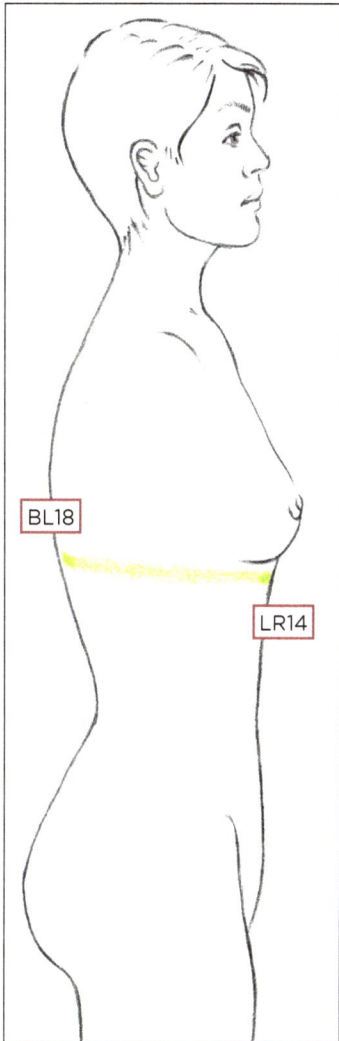

BL18

LR14

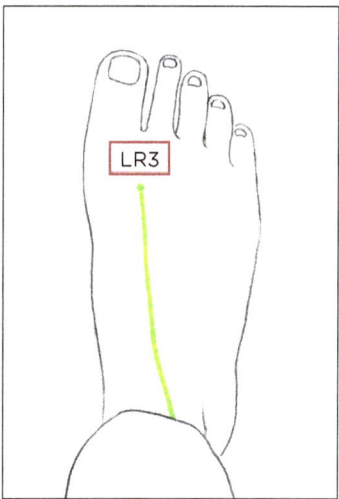

LR3

GB37

ST42

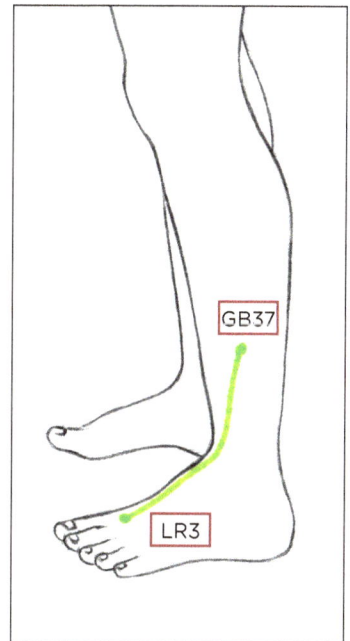

GB37

LR3

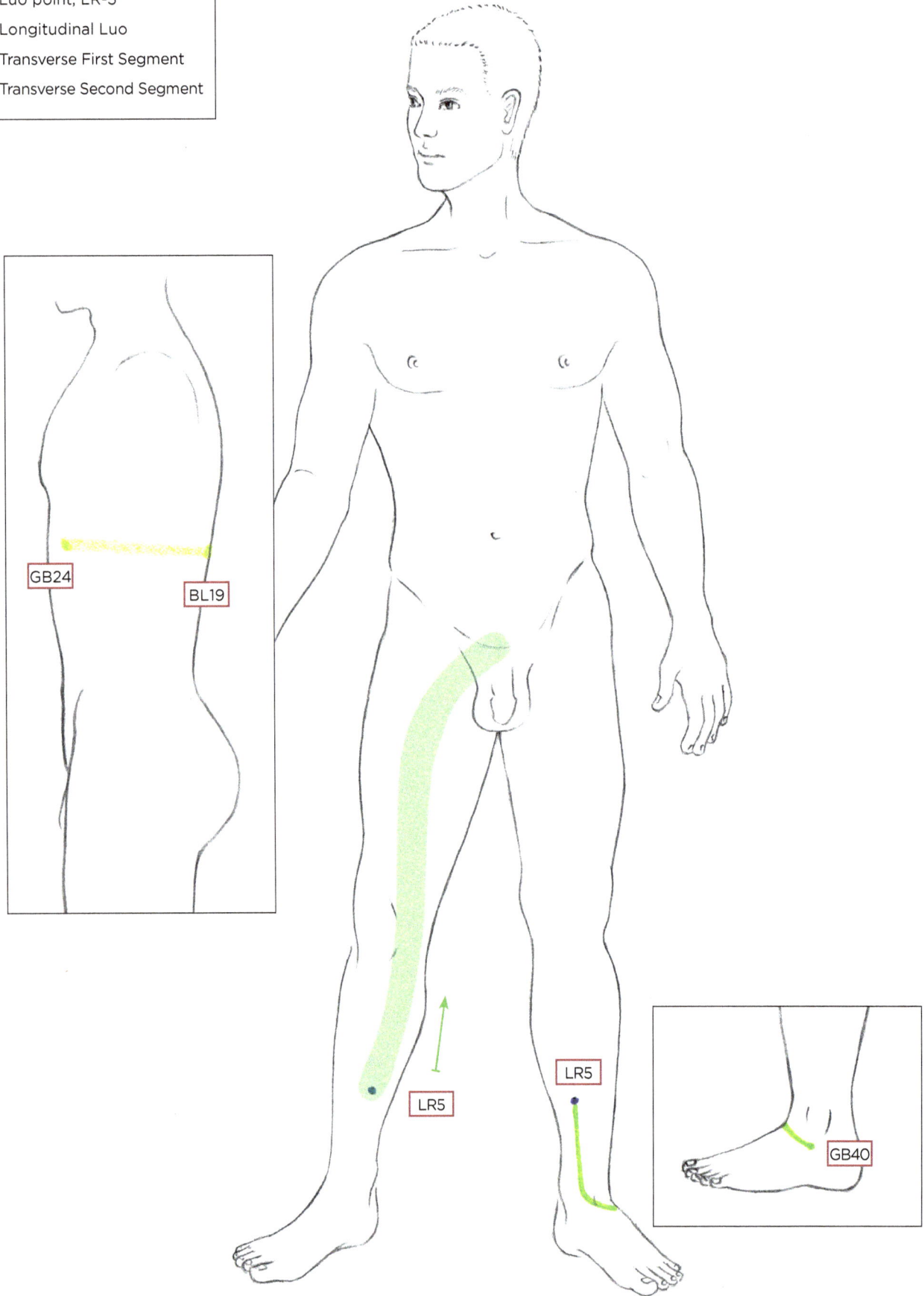

Liver Luo Channel

Luo point, LR-5
Longitudinal Luo
Transverse First Segment
Transverse Second Segment

LUO

GB24

BL19

LR5

LR5

GB40

26

	Luo point, CV-15
	Luo trajectory

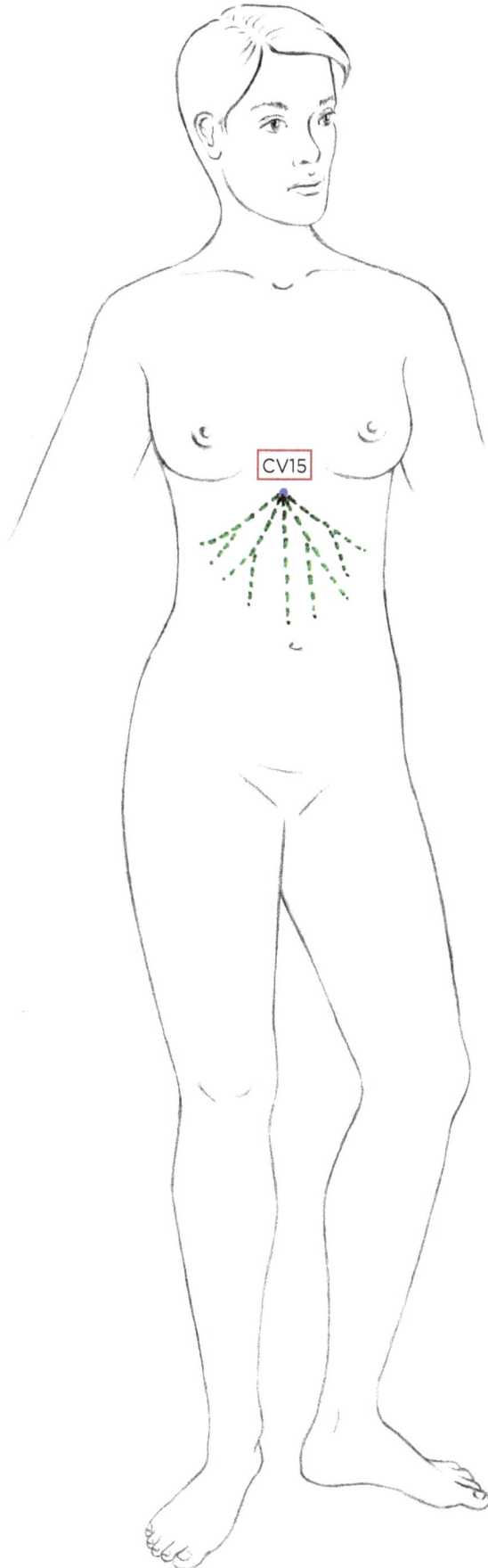

CV15

Du Luo Channel

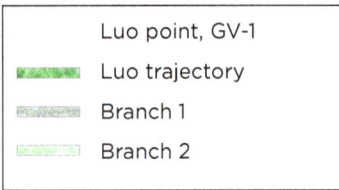

- ⬤ Luo point, GV-1
- ▬ Luo trajectory
- ▬ Branch 1
- ▬ Branch 2

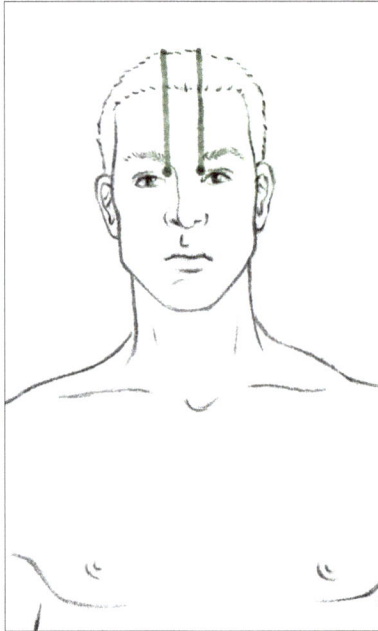

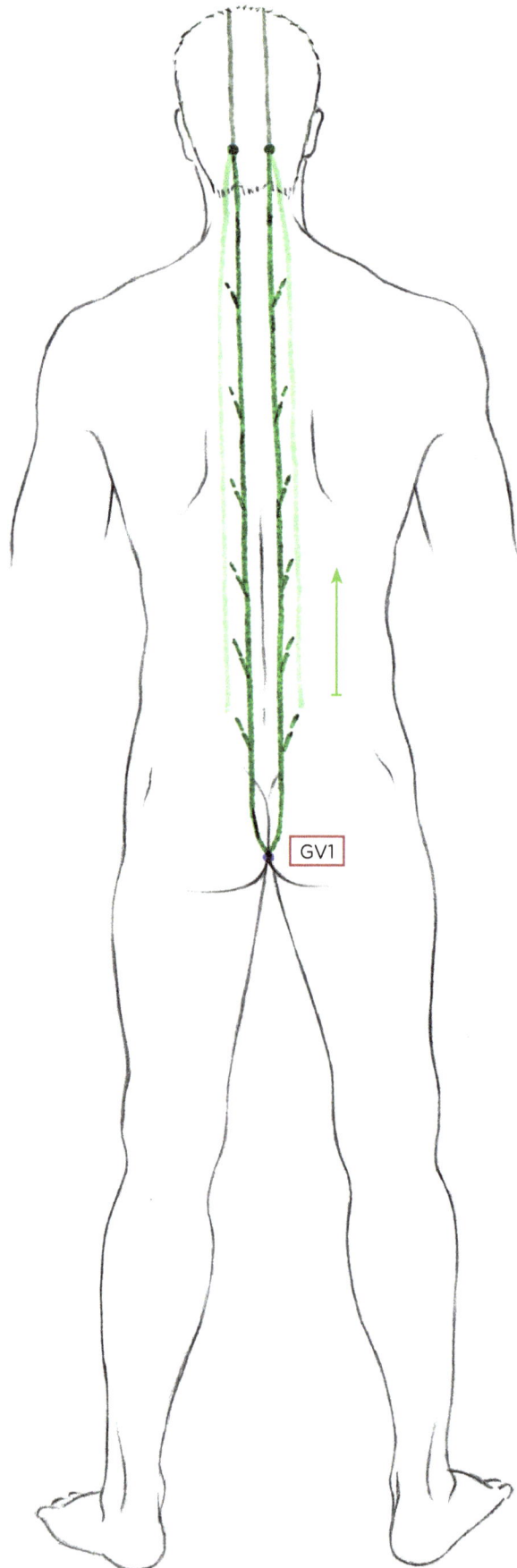

GV1

Great Luo of the Spleen

	Luo point, GB-22
▬	Longitudinal Luo

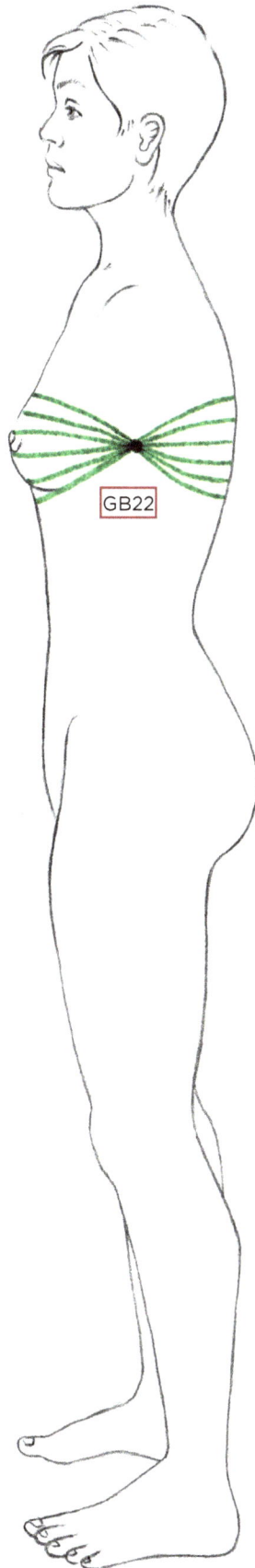

GB22

Great Luo of the Stomach

	Su Wen trajectory

CV12

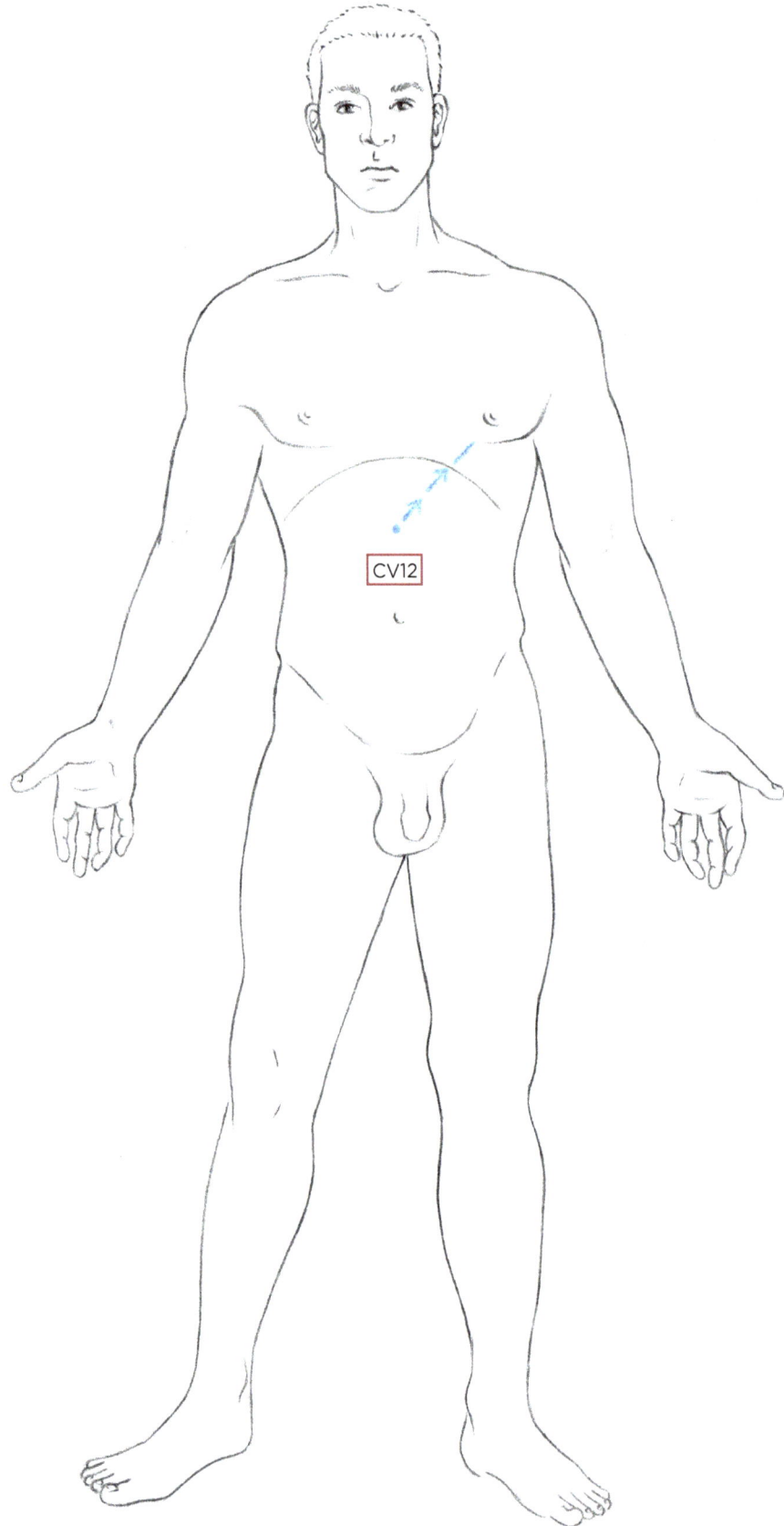

This channel has no points and extends from the solar plexus to the heart.

30

The Divergent Channels

Bladder Divergent Channel

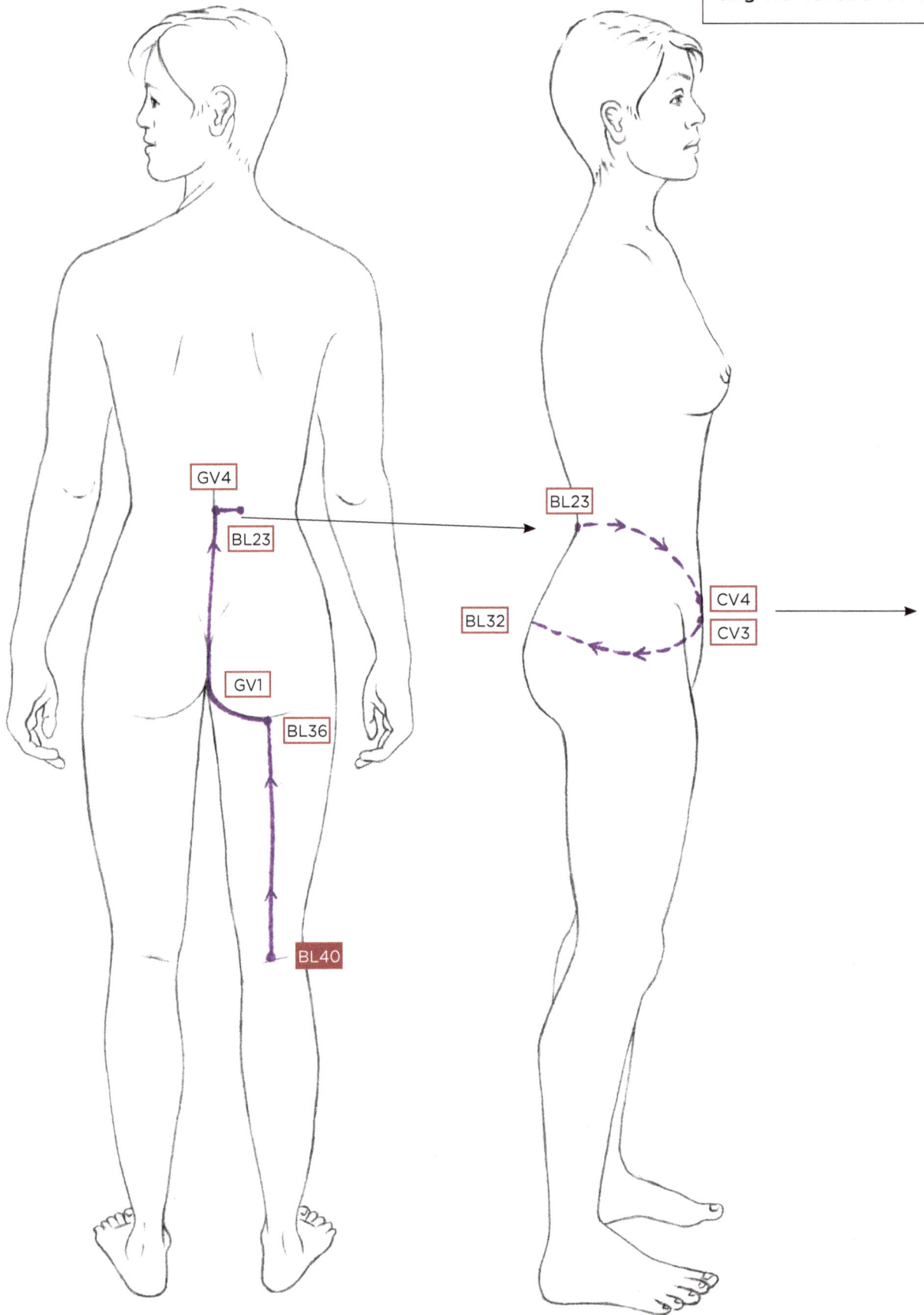

Confluence points: ▮
Trajectory points: ▢
Jing-Well for SDS: BL-67

GV4
BL23
GV1
BL36
BL40

BL23
BL32
CV4
CV3

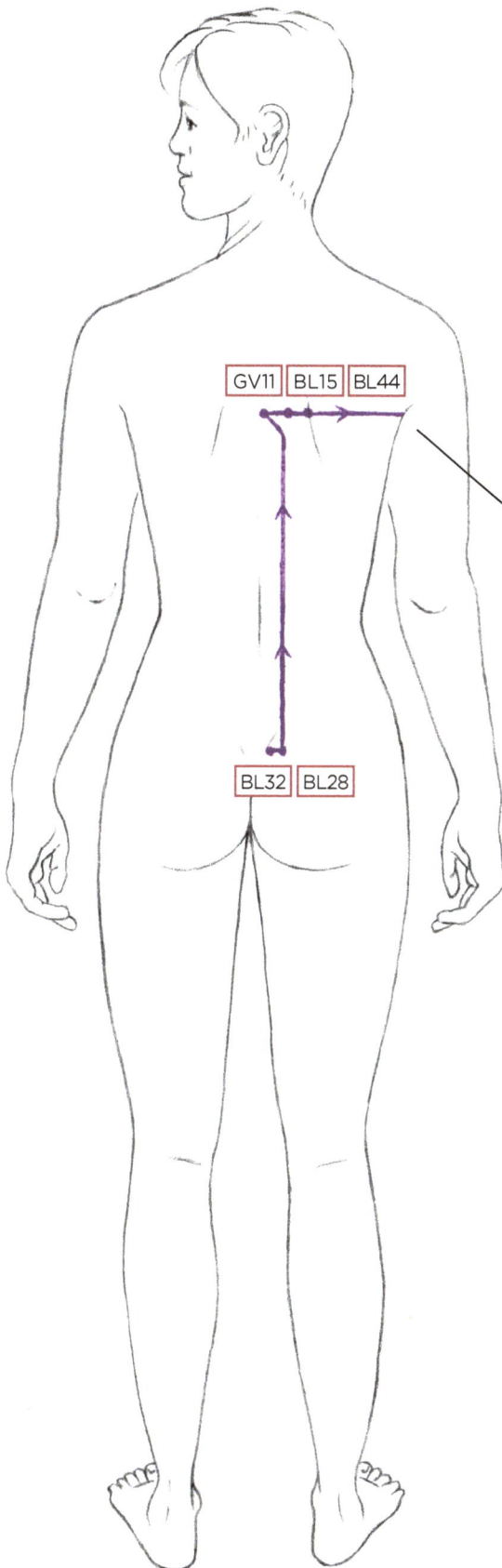

GV11 | BL15 | BL44

BL32 | BL28

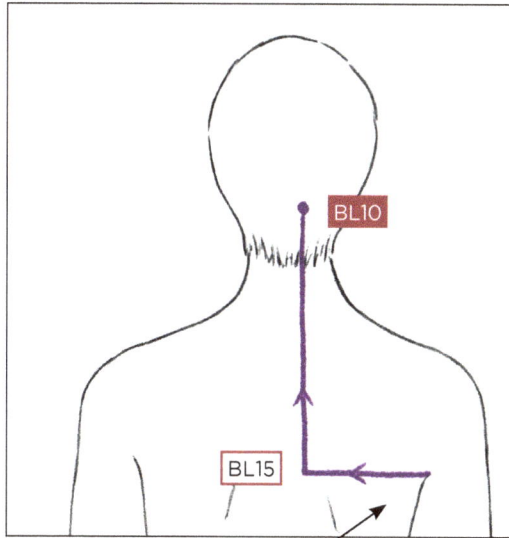

BL10

BL15

CV17

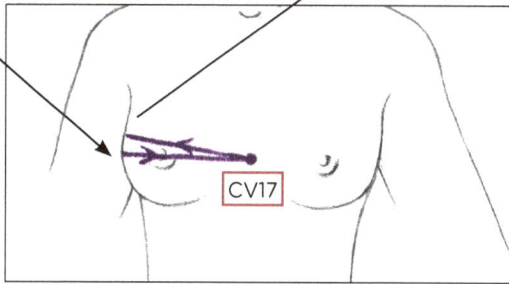

***Tai Yang* Cutaneous region**

This region wraps around the chest at the level of GB-22, CV-17 and BL-17, skirting under the inferior angle of the scapula. In my experience, it also extends from that band, medial to the medial border of the scapula to GB-21.

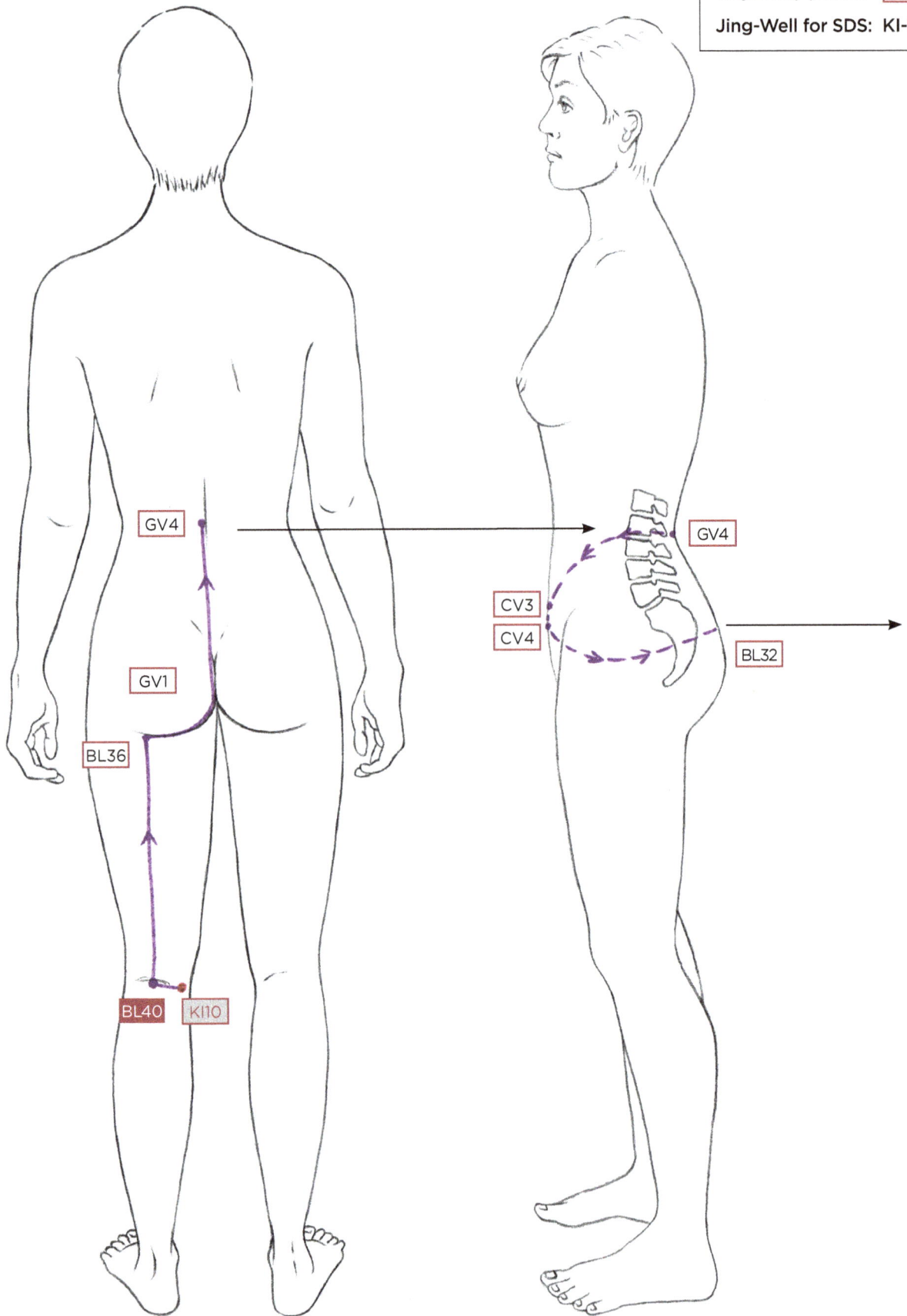

Kidney Divergent Channel

DIVERGENT

GV4

GV4

CV3

CV4

BL32

GV1

BL36

BL40   KI10

34

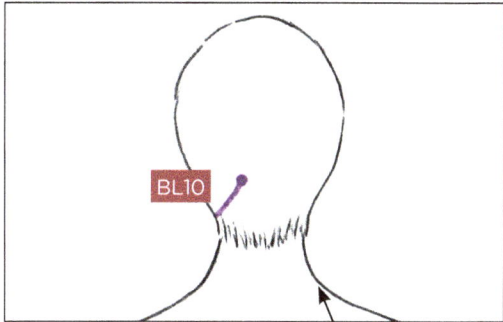

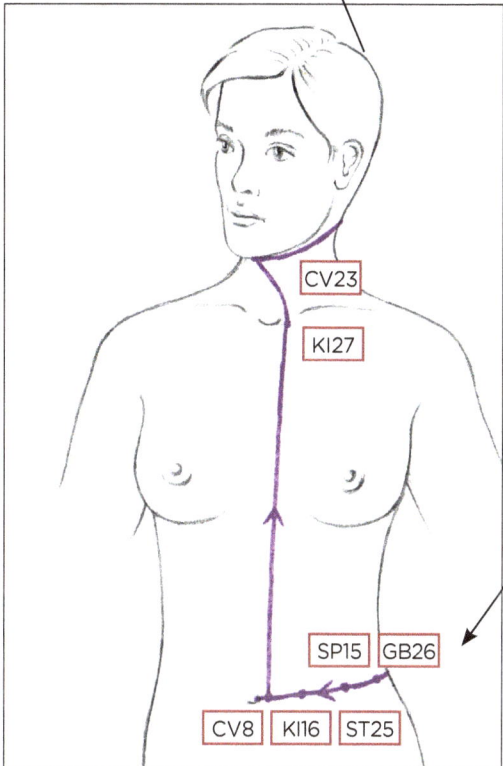

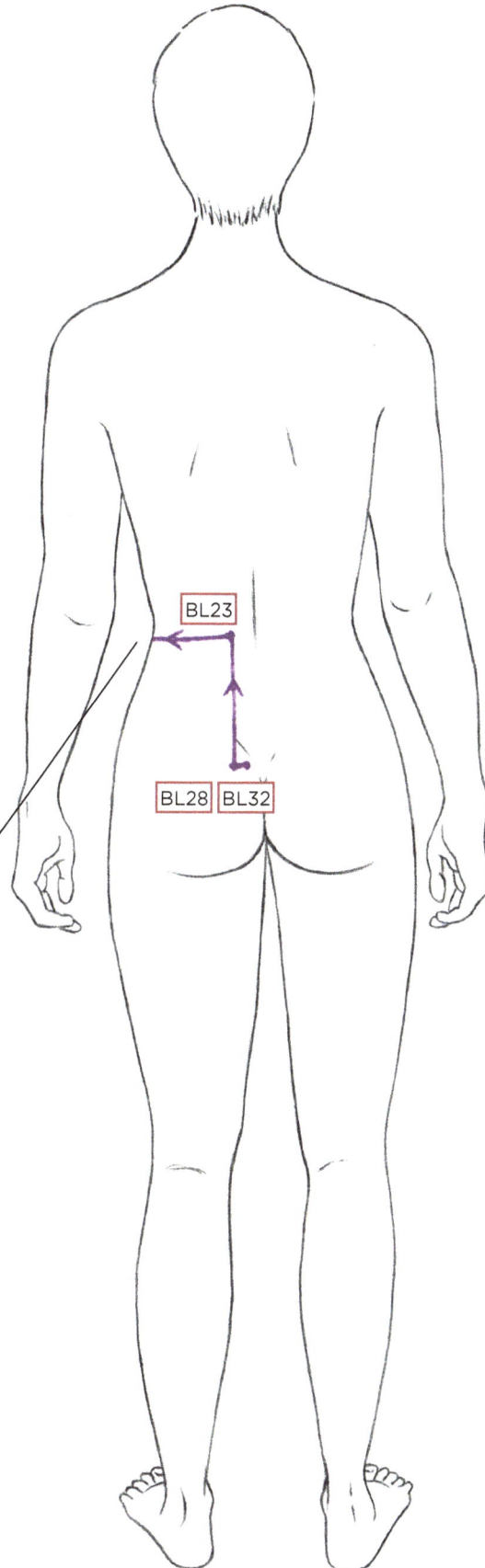

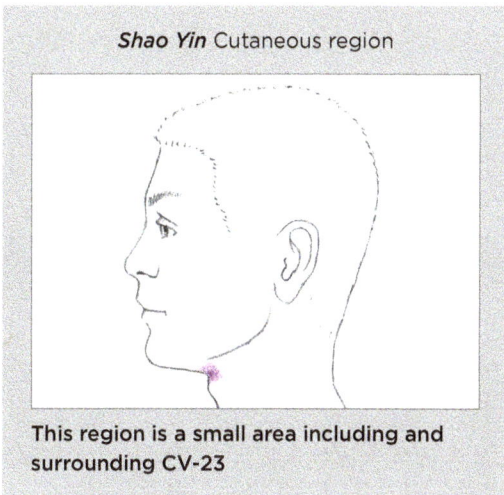

Shao Yin Cutaneous region

This region is a small area including and surrounding CV-23

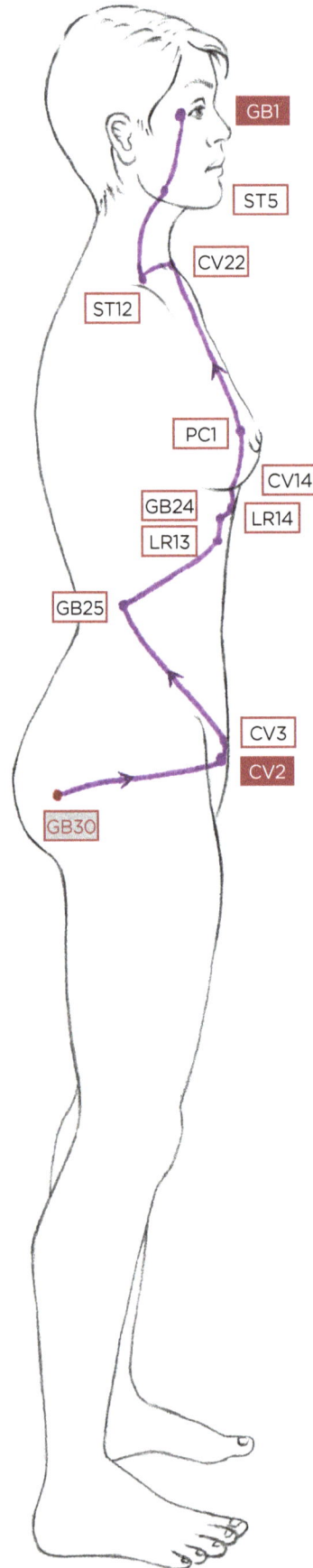

Gallbladder Divergent Channel

Confluence points: ▮
Opening Points: ▮
Trajectory points: ☐
Jing-Well for SDS: GB-44

GB1
ST5
CV22
ST12
PC1
CV14
GB24
LR14
LR13
GB25
CV3
CV2
GB30

Shao Yang Cutaneous region

This region is a band that extends from the area of GB-25 and LR-13 to CV-3 and CV-2. Another part is the tight area around and including TH-16 and GB-12.

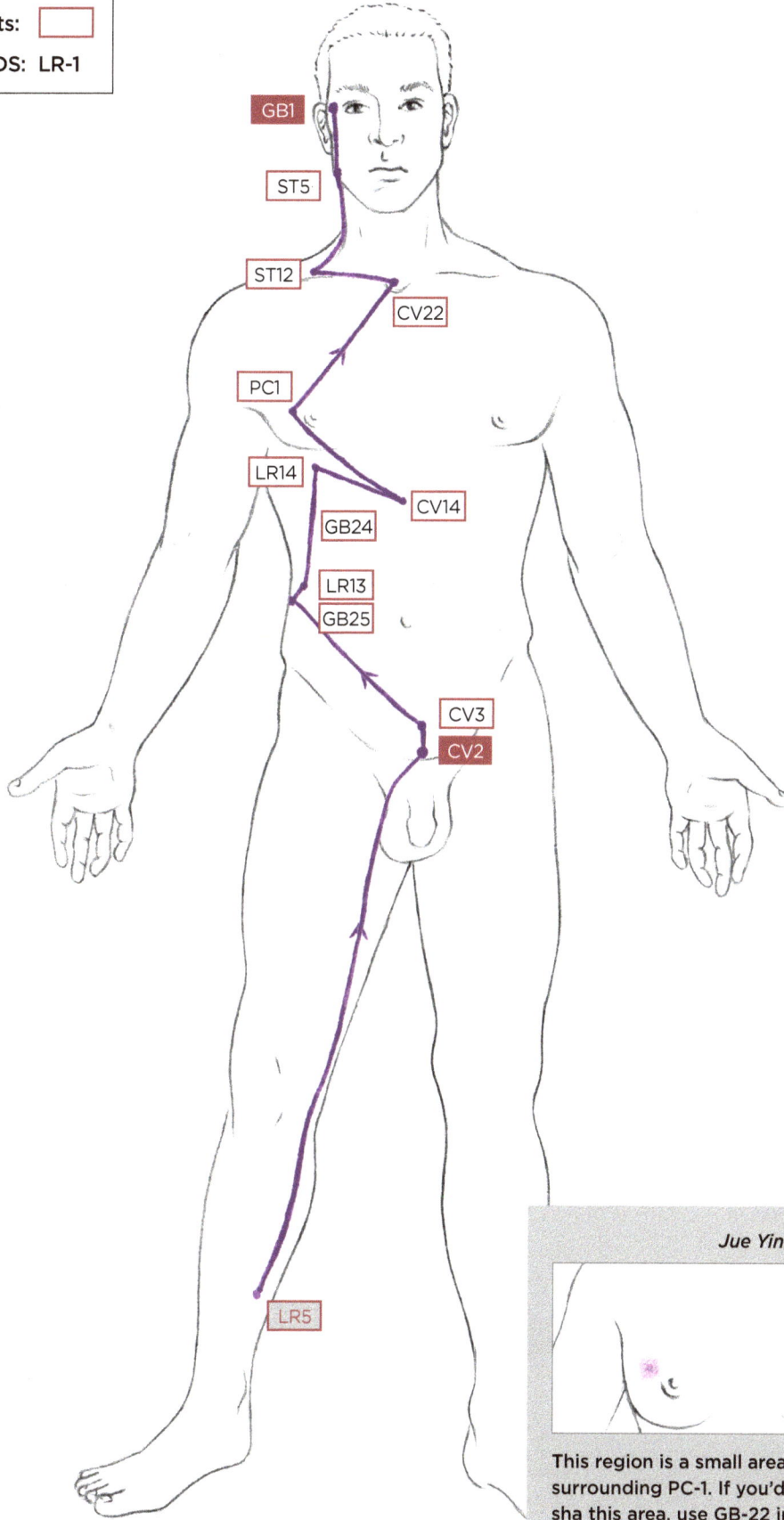

Confluence points: ▮
Opening Points: ▮
Trajectory points: ▯
Jing-Well for SDS: LR-1

GB1
ST5
ST12
CV22
PC1
LR14
CV14
GB24
LR13
GB25
CV3
CV2
LR5

DIVERGENT

Jue Yin

This region is a small area including and surrounding PC-1. If you'd prefer not to gua sha this area, use GB-22 instead.

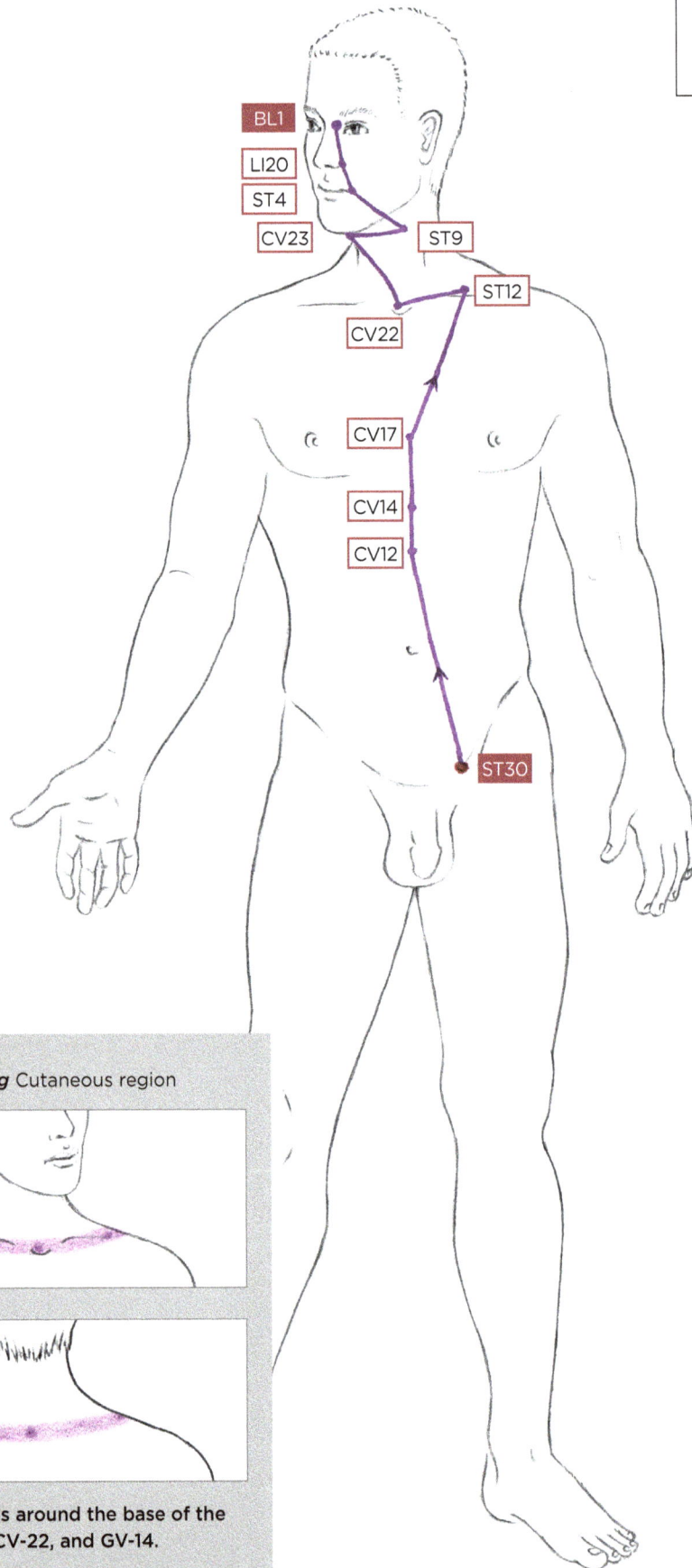

Stomach Divergent Channel

DIVERGENT

BL1
LI20
ST4
CV23
ST9
ST12
CV22
CV17
CV14
CV12
ST30

Yang Ming Cutaneous region

This region wraps around the base of the throat, through CV-22, and GV-14.

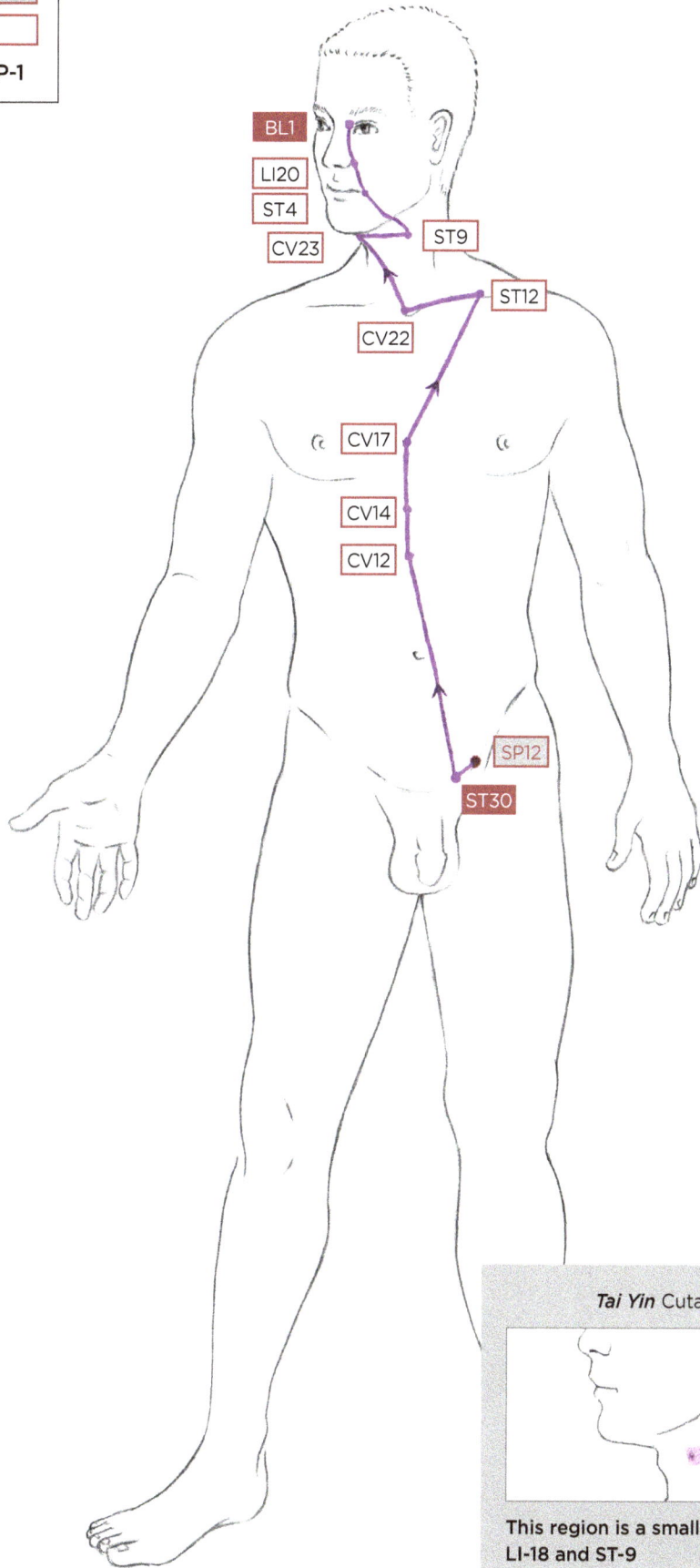

Confluence points:

Opening Points:

Trajectory points:

Jing-Well for SDS: SP-1

BL1

LI20

ST4

CV23

ST9

ST12

CV22

CV17

CV14

CV12

SP12

ST30

DIVERGENT

Tai Yin Cutaneous region

This region is a small area of tightness near LI-18 and ST-9

Small Intestine Divergent Channel

DIVERGENT

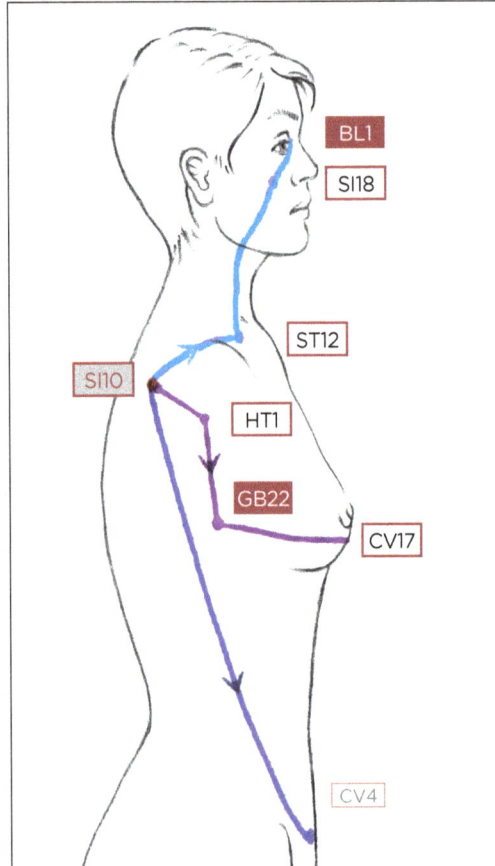

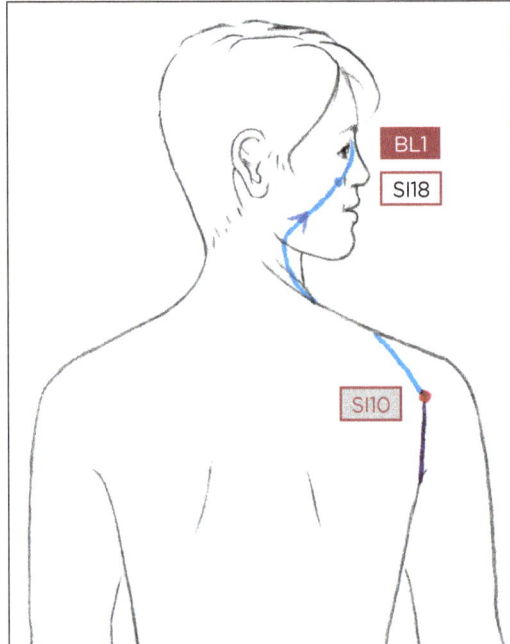

Tai Yang Cutaneous region

This region wraps around the chest at the level of GB-22, CV-17 and BL-17, skirting under the inferior angle of the scapula. In my experience, it also extends from that band, medial to the medial border of the scapula to GB-21.

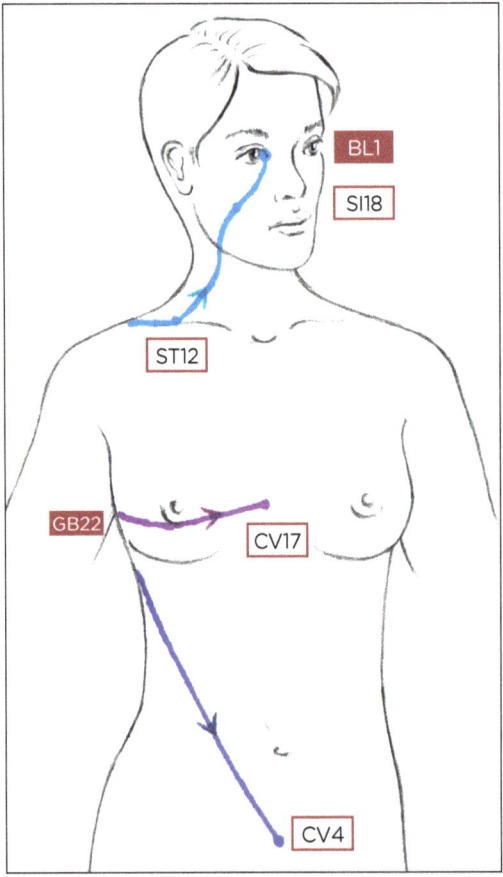

Confluence points:	
Opening Points:	
Trajectory points:	
Jing-Well for SDS:	HT-9

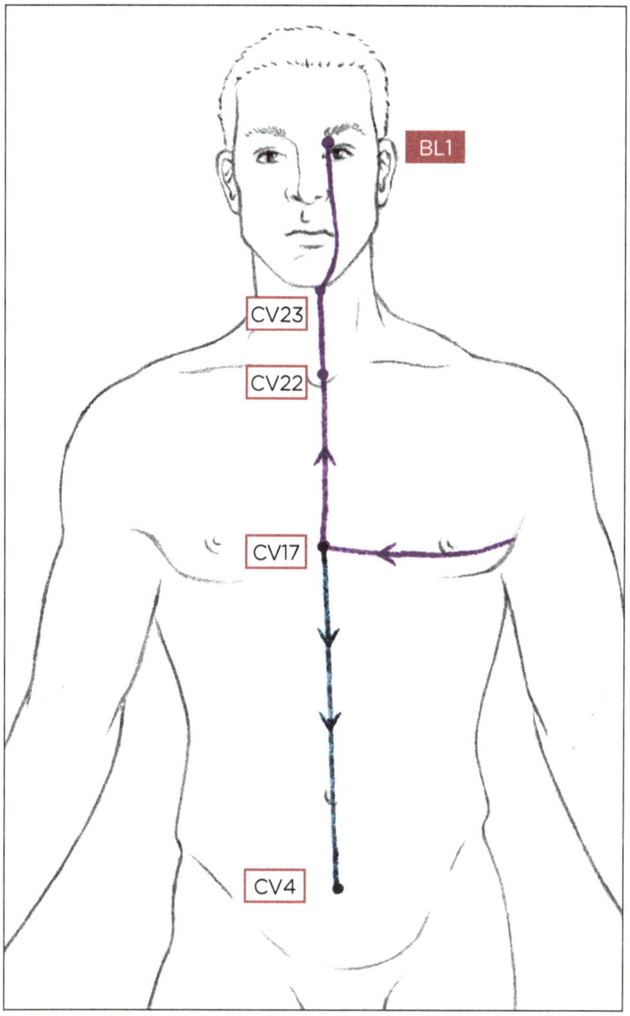

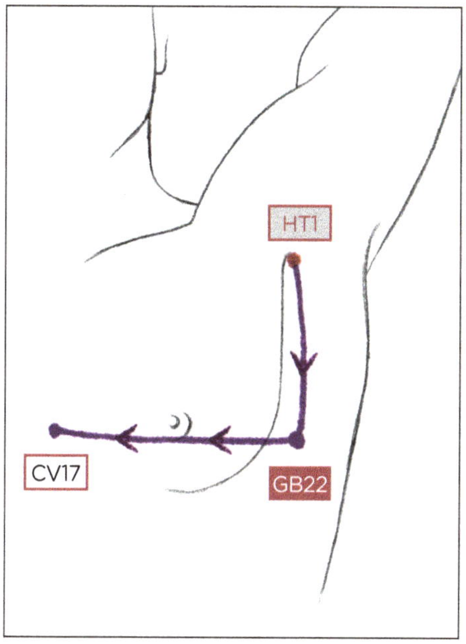

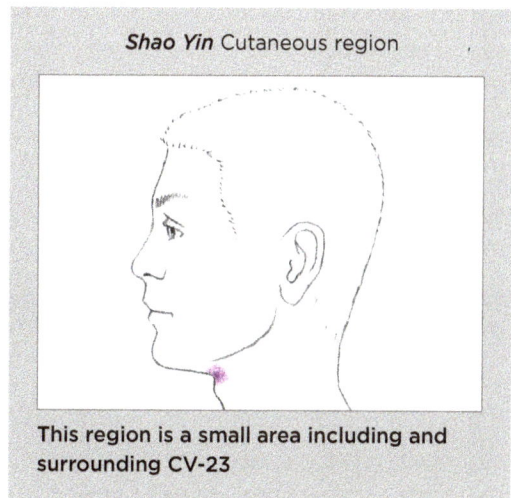

Shao Yin Cutaneous region

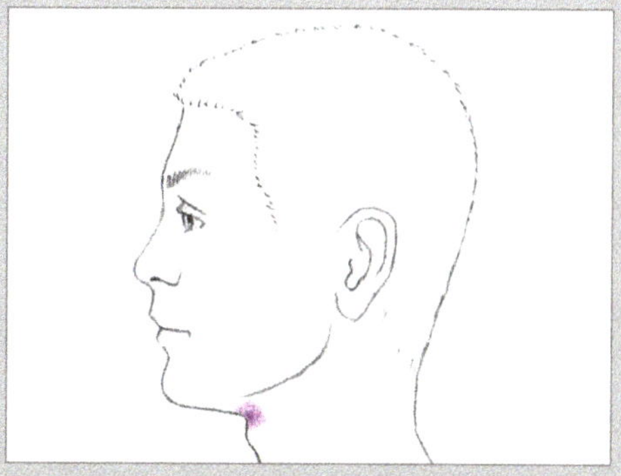

This region is a small area including and surrounding CV-23

Triple Heater Divergent Channel

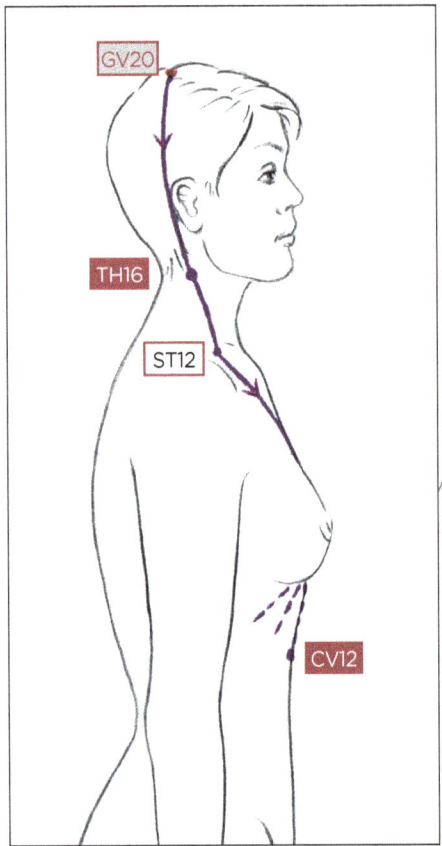

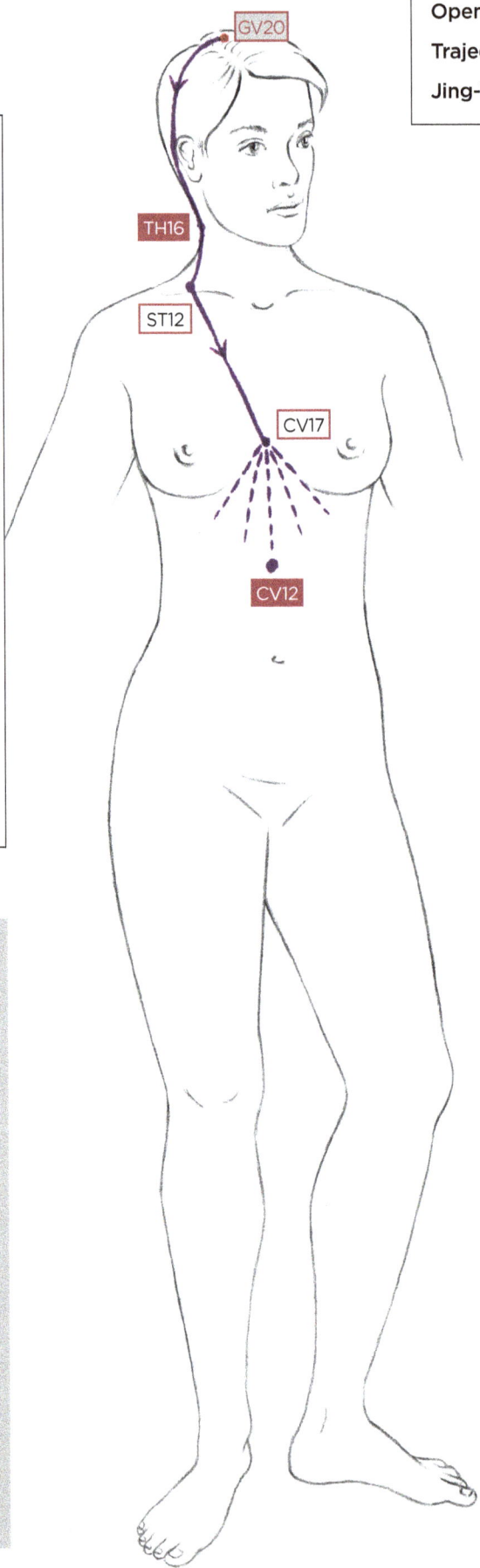

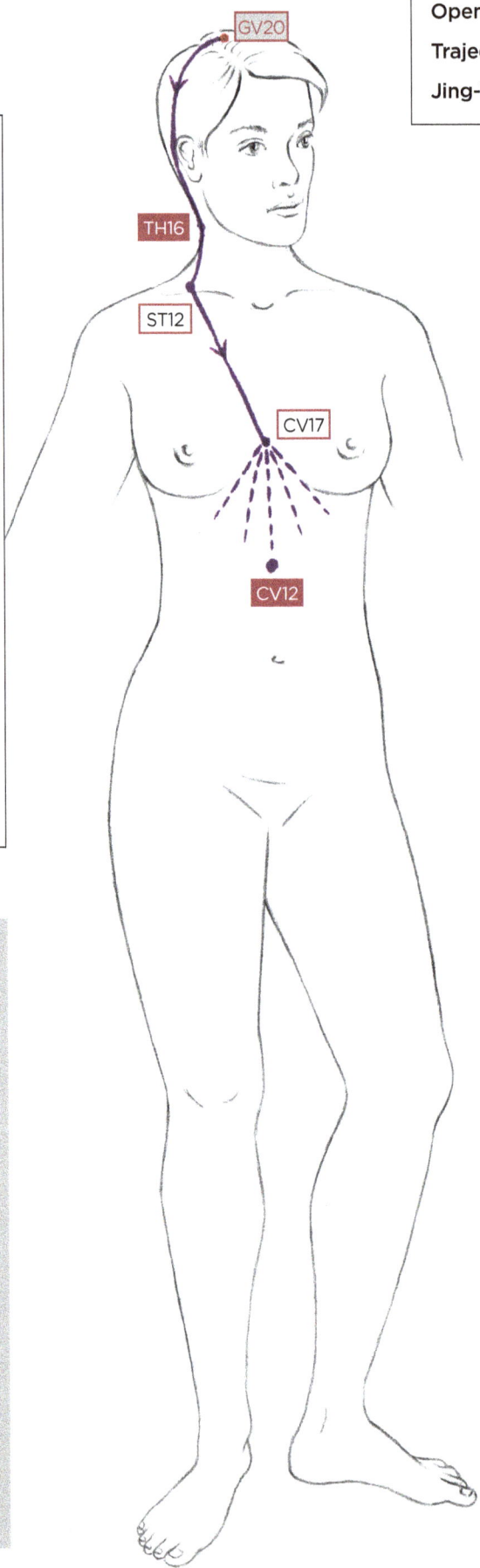 labels: GV20, TH16, ST12, CV17, CV12

Shao Yang Cutaneous region

This region is a band that extends from the area of GB-25 and LR-13 to CV-3 and CV-2. Another part is the tight area around and including TH-16 and GB-12.

DIVERGENT

Confluence points:
Opening Points:
Trajectory points:
Jing-Well for SDS: PC-9

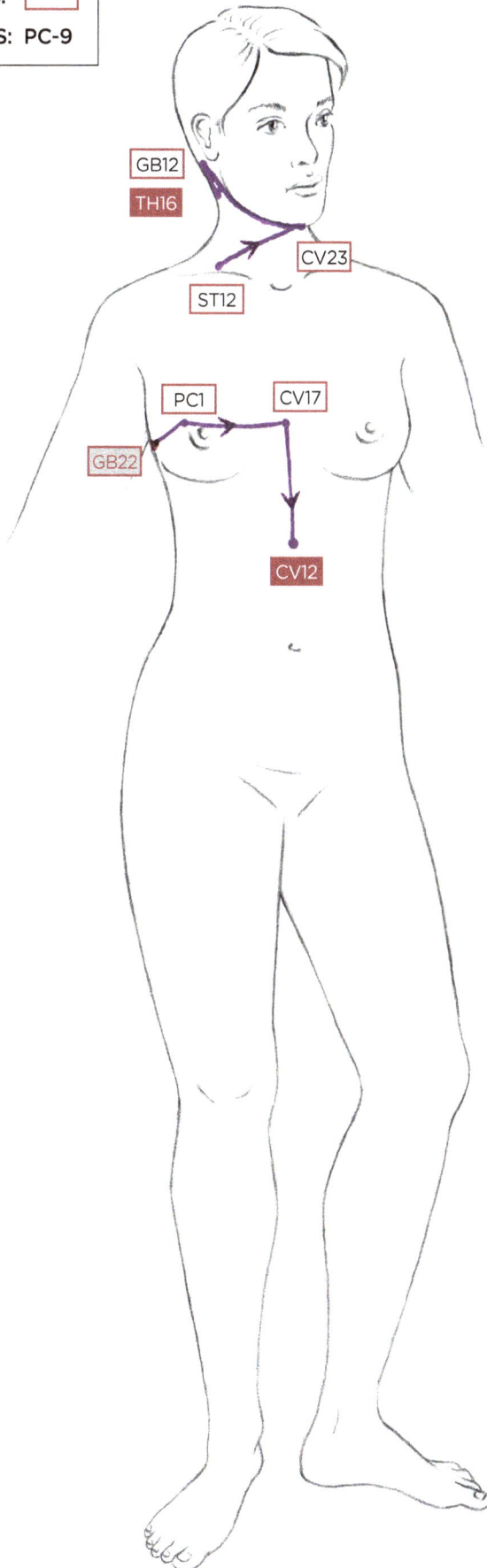

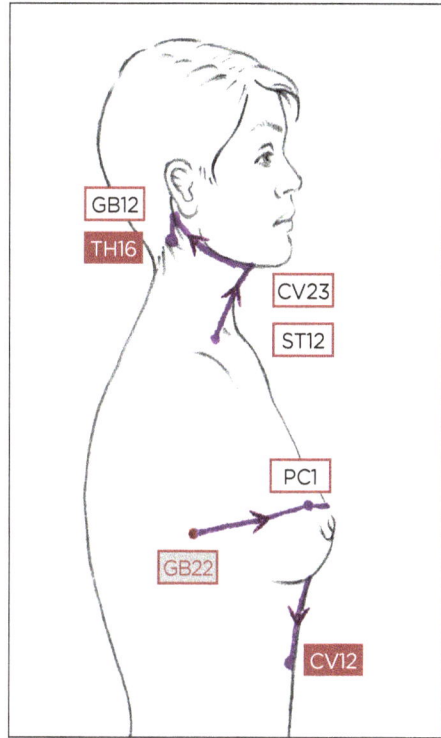

DIVERGENT

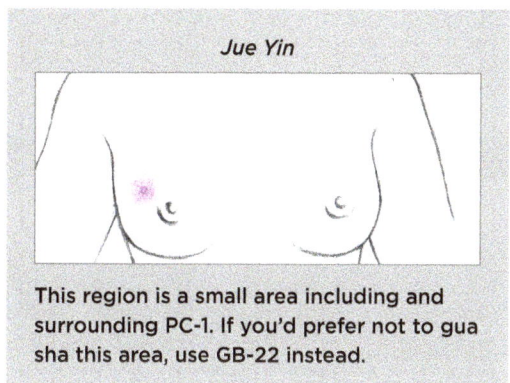

Jue Yin

This region is a small area including and surrounding PC-1. If you'd prefer not to gua sha this area, use GB-22 instead.

Large Intestine Divergent Channel

Confluence points:
Opening Points:
Trajectory points:
Jing-Well for SDS: LI-1

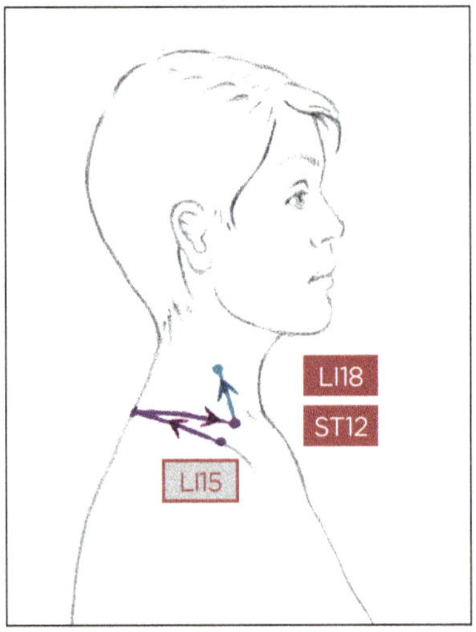
LI18
ST12
LI15

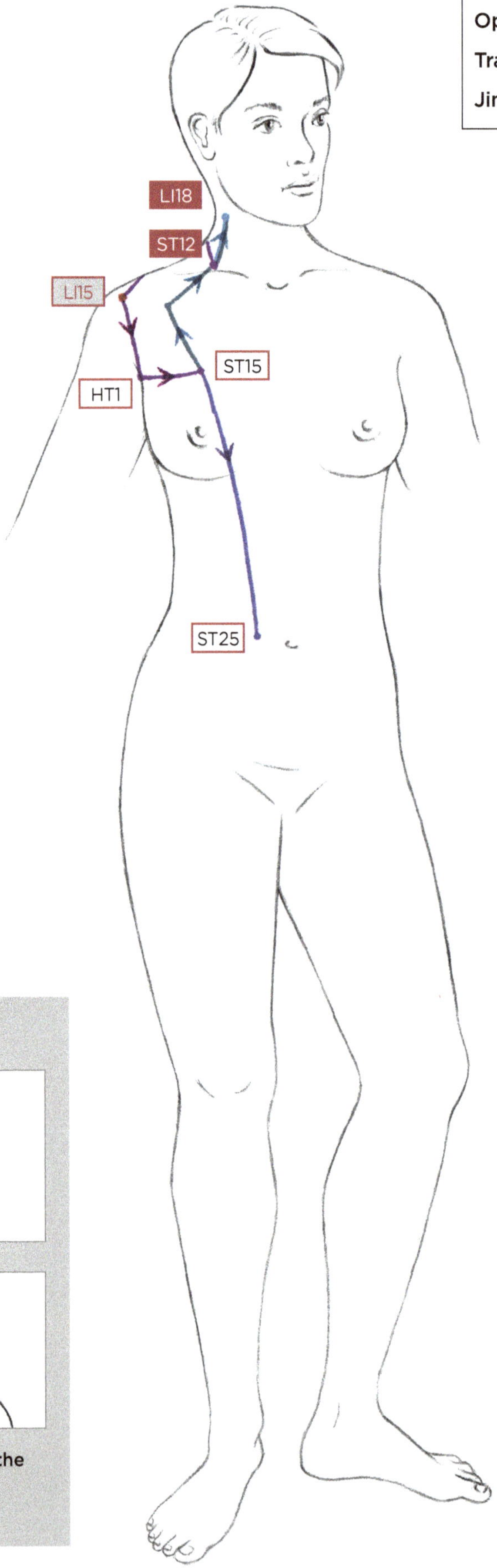
LI18
ST12
LI15
ST15
HT1
ST25

Yang Ming Cutaneous region

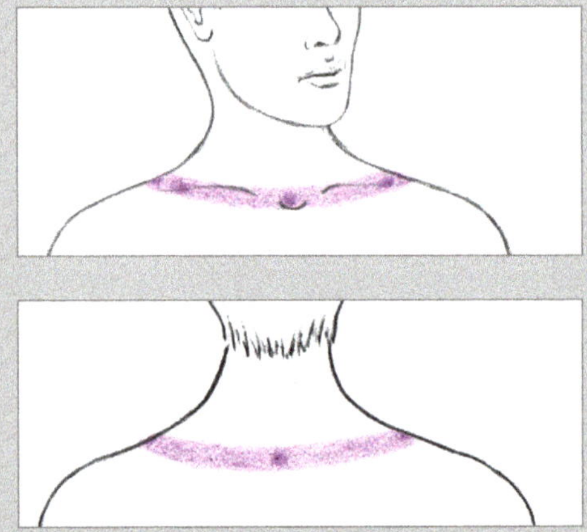

This region wraps around the base of the throat, through CV-22, and GV-14.

Confluence points:
Opening Points:
Trajectory points:
Jing-Well for SDS: LU-11

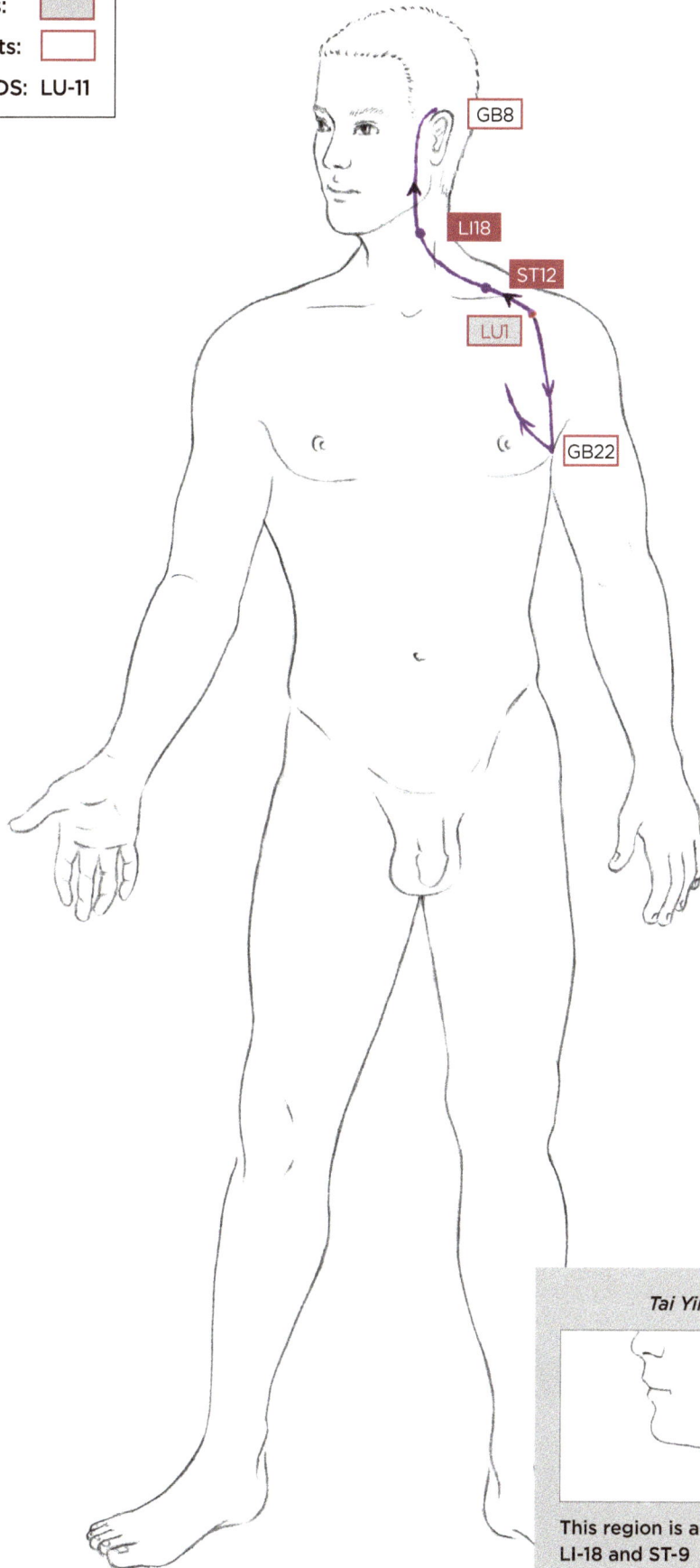

GB8

LI18

ST12

LU1

GB22

DIVERGENT

Tai Yin Cutaneous region

This region is a small area of tightness near LI-18 and ST-9

The Eight Extraordinary Channels

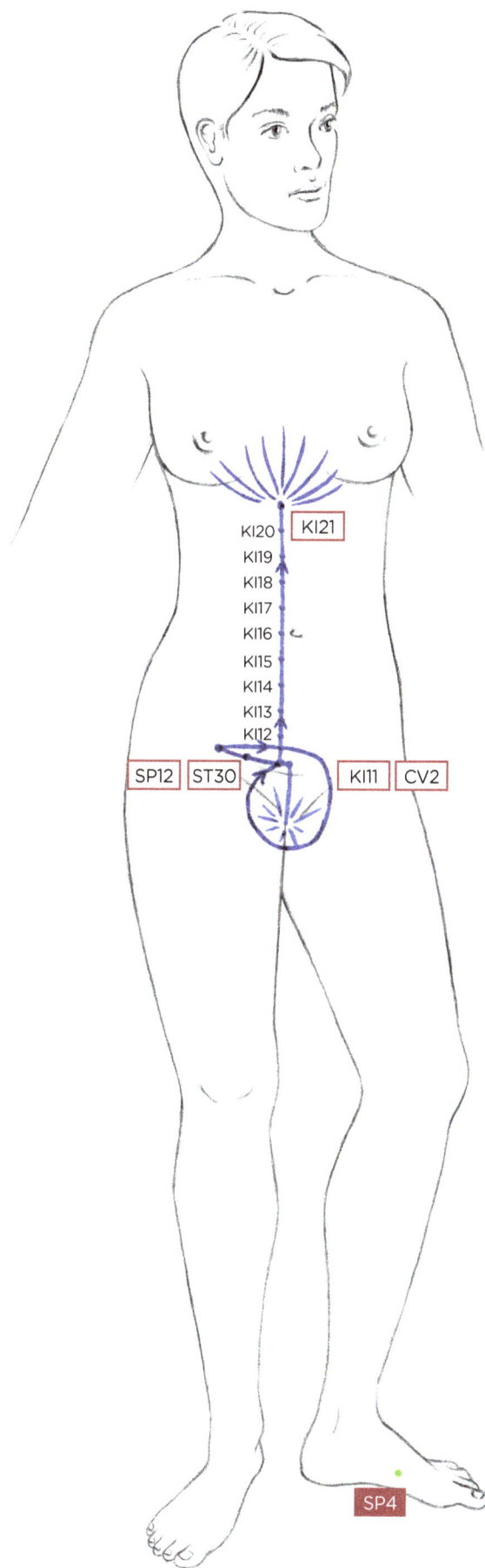

KI20
KI19
KI18
KI17
KI16
KI15
KI14
KI13
KI12

KI21

SP12 ST30   KI11 CV2

SP4

Chong Mai

Second Trajectory

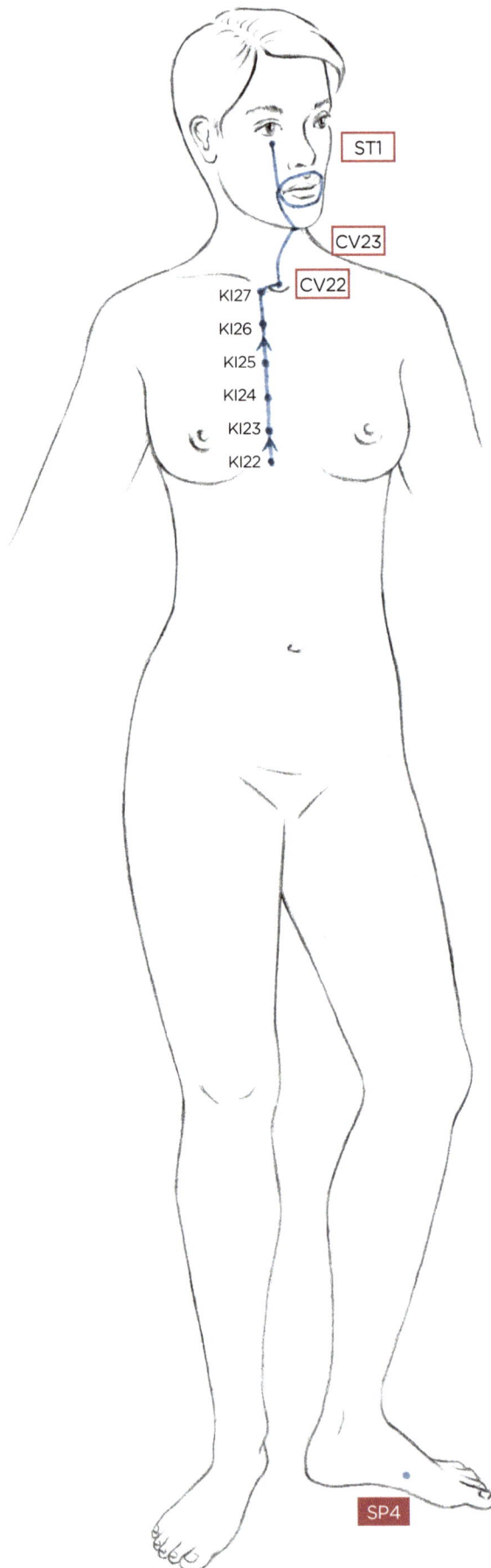

ST1

CV23

CV22

KI27
KI26
KI25
KI24
KI23
KI22

SP4

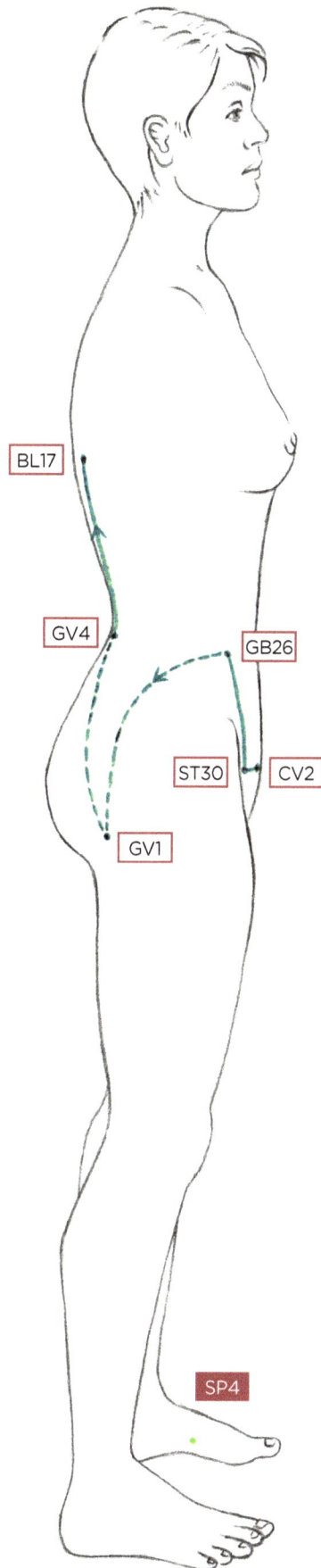

8 EXTRA

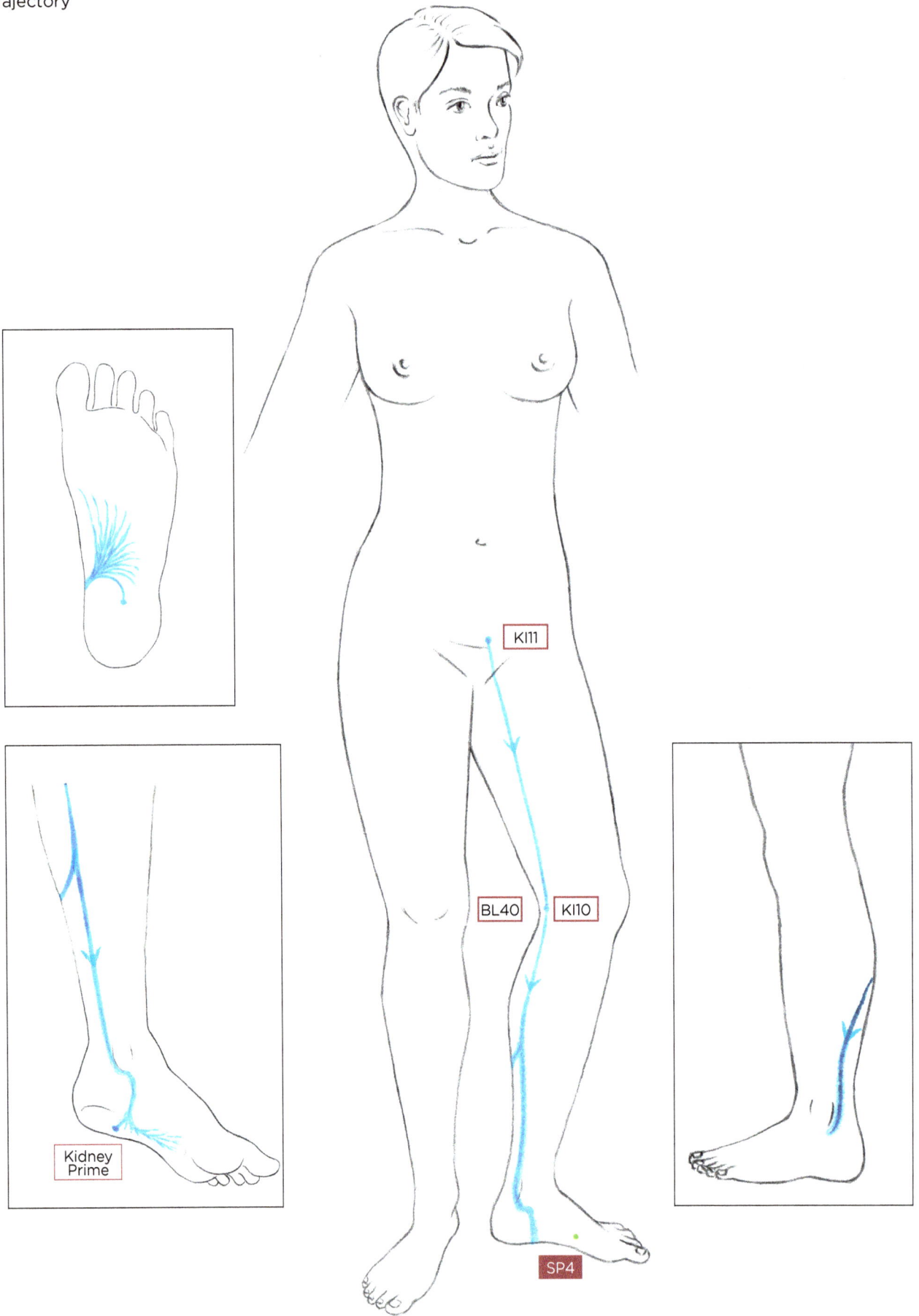

Chong Mai

Fourth Trajectory

KI11

BL40   KI10

Kidney
Prime

SP4

50

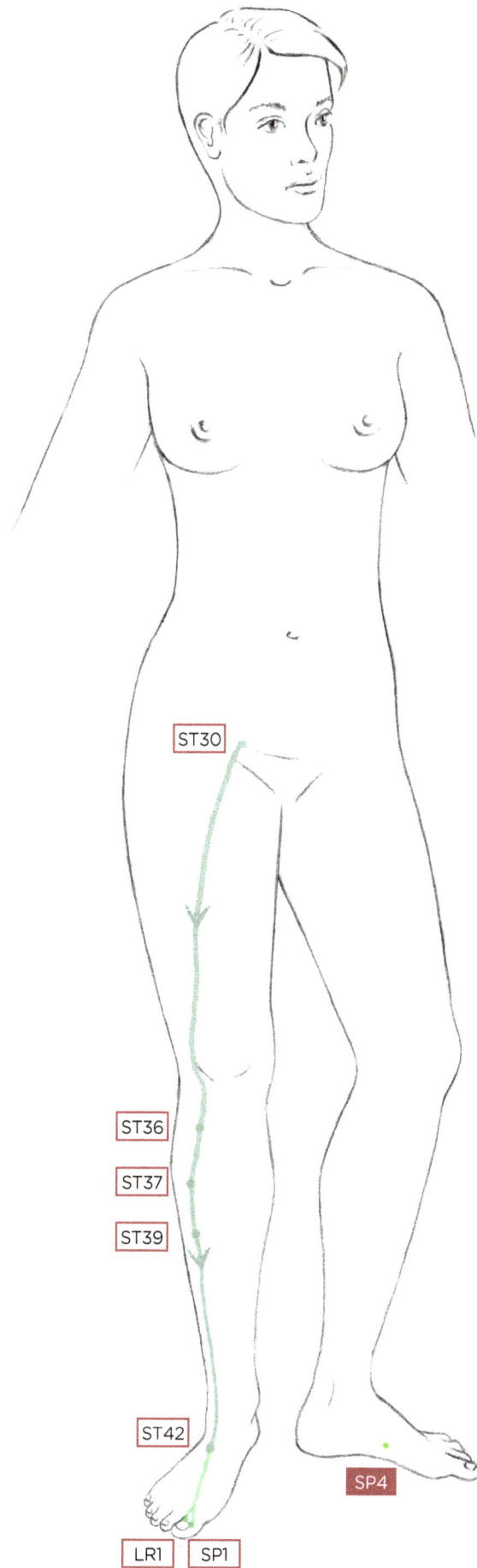

ST30

ST36

ST37

ST39

ST42

SP4

LR1   SP1

Ren Mai

ST1

ST4

CV24

CV23

CV22

CV2

CV1

GV14

LU7

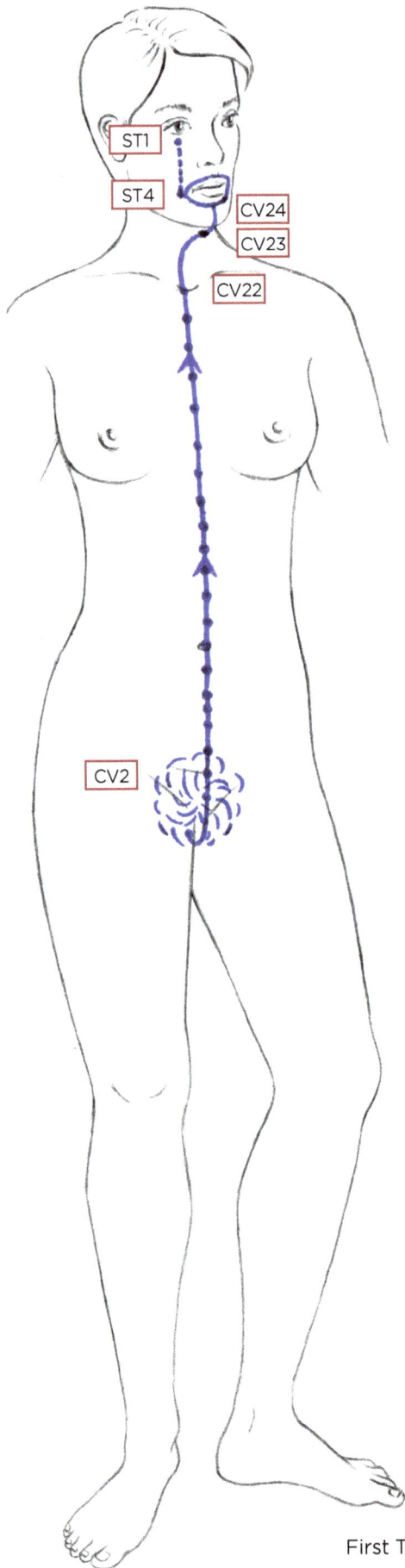

First Trajectory

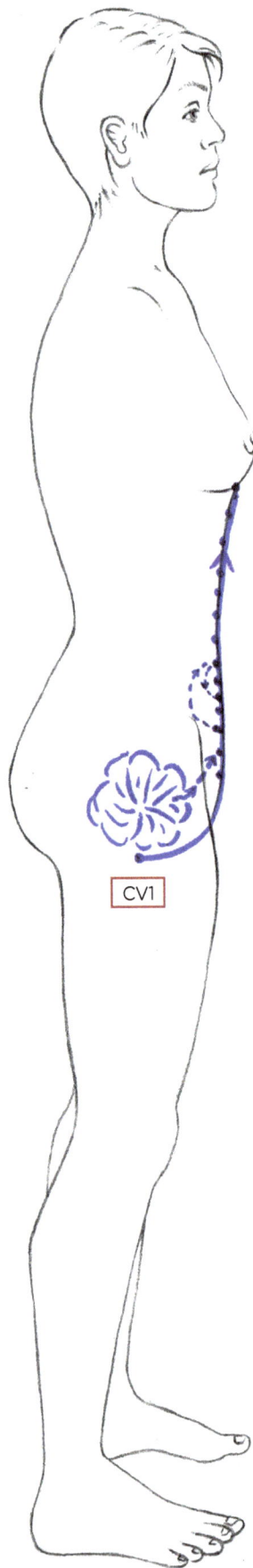

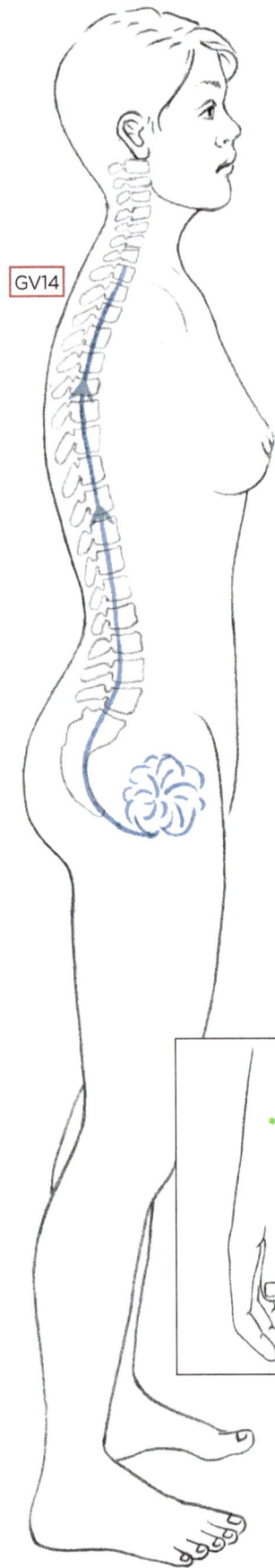

Second Trajectory

52

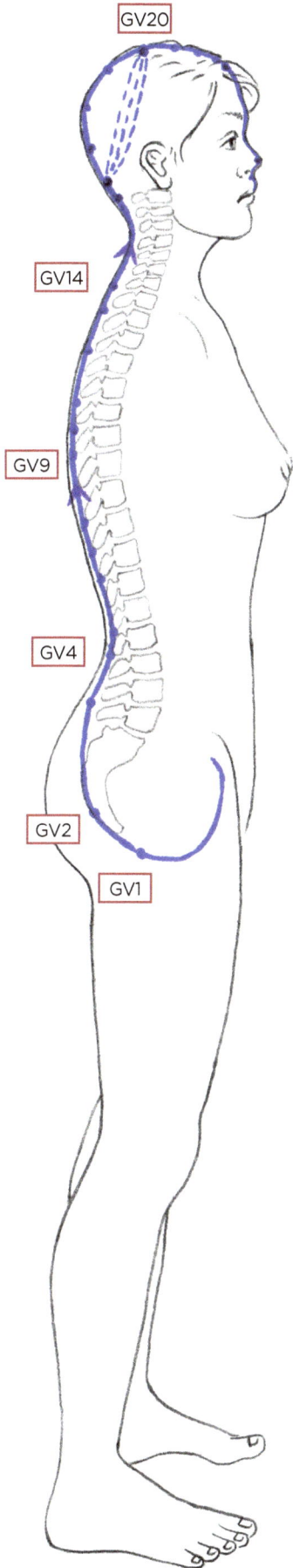

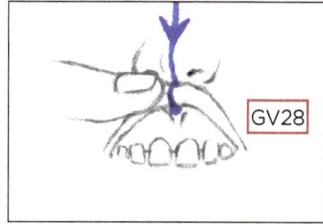

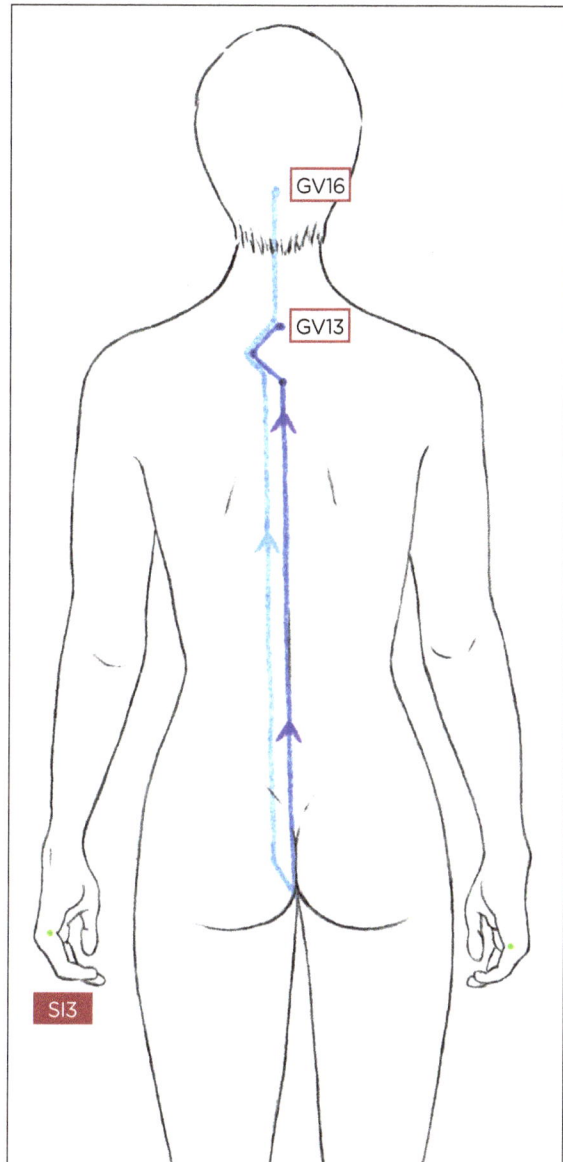

GV20

GV14

GV9

GV4

GV2

GV1

GV28

GV16

GV13

SI3

A and B

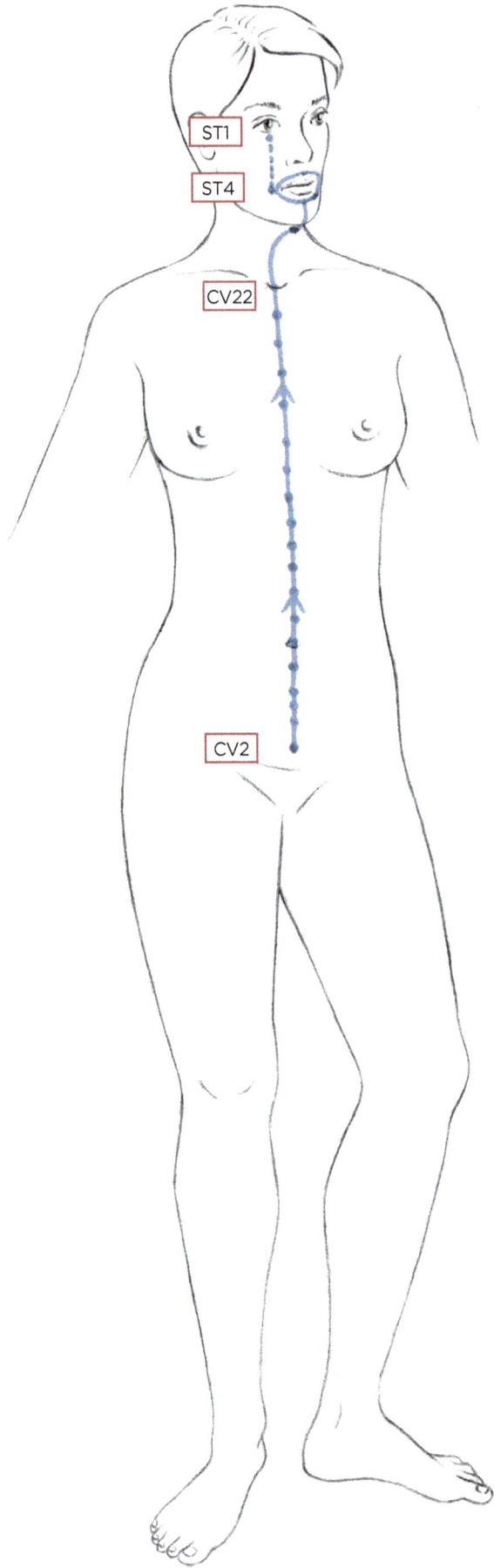

ST1

ST4

CV22

CV2

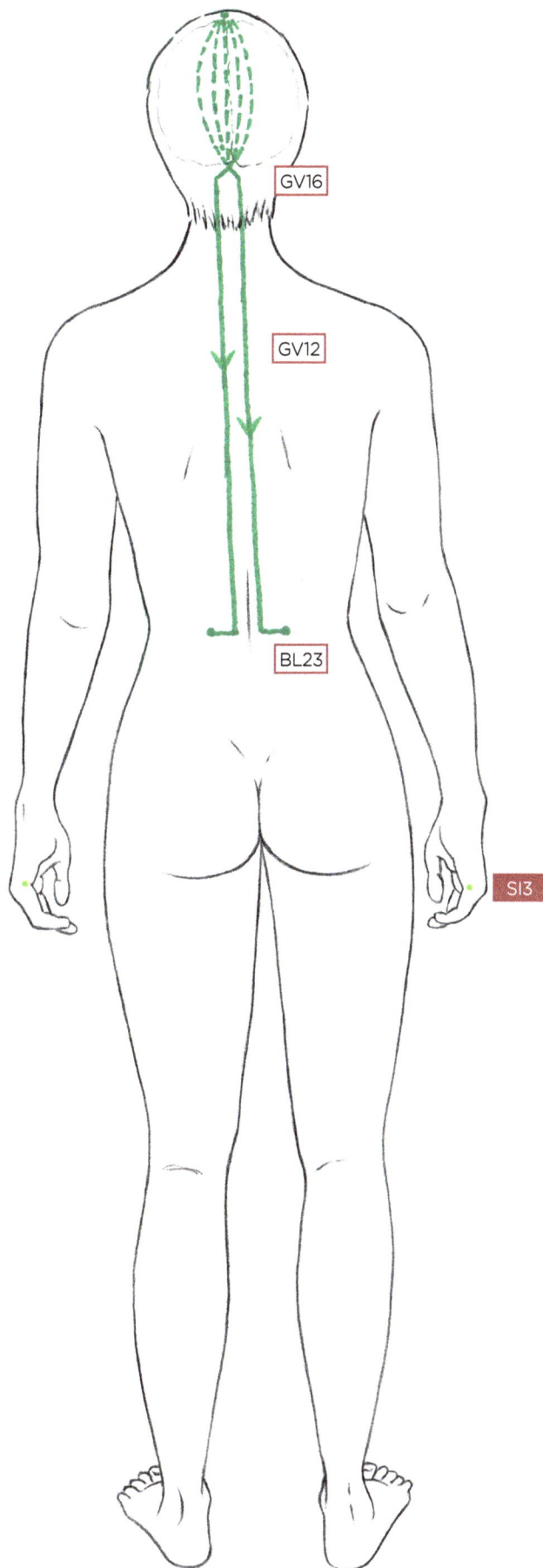

GV16

GV12

BL23

SI3

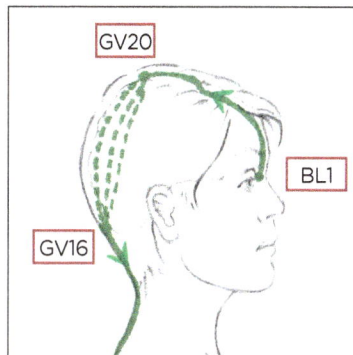

GV20

BL1

GV16

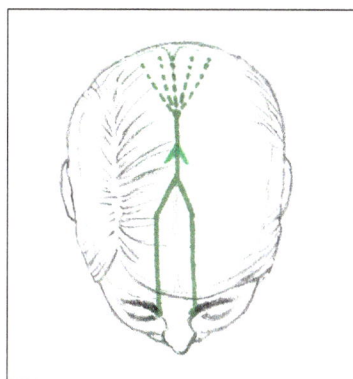

8 EXTRA

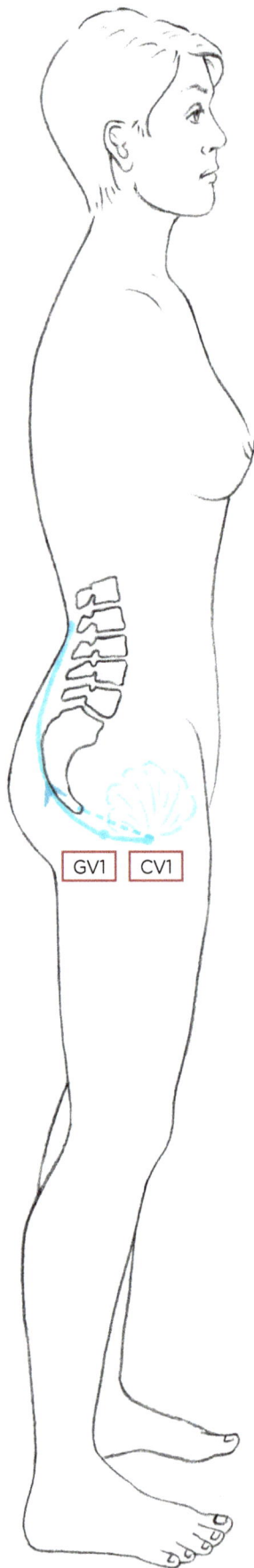

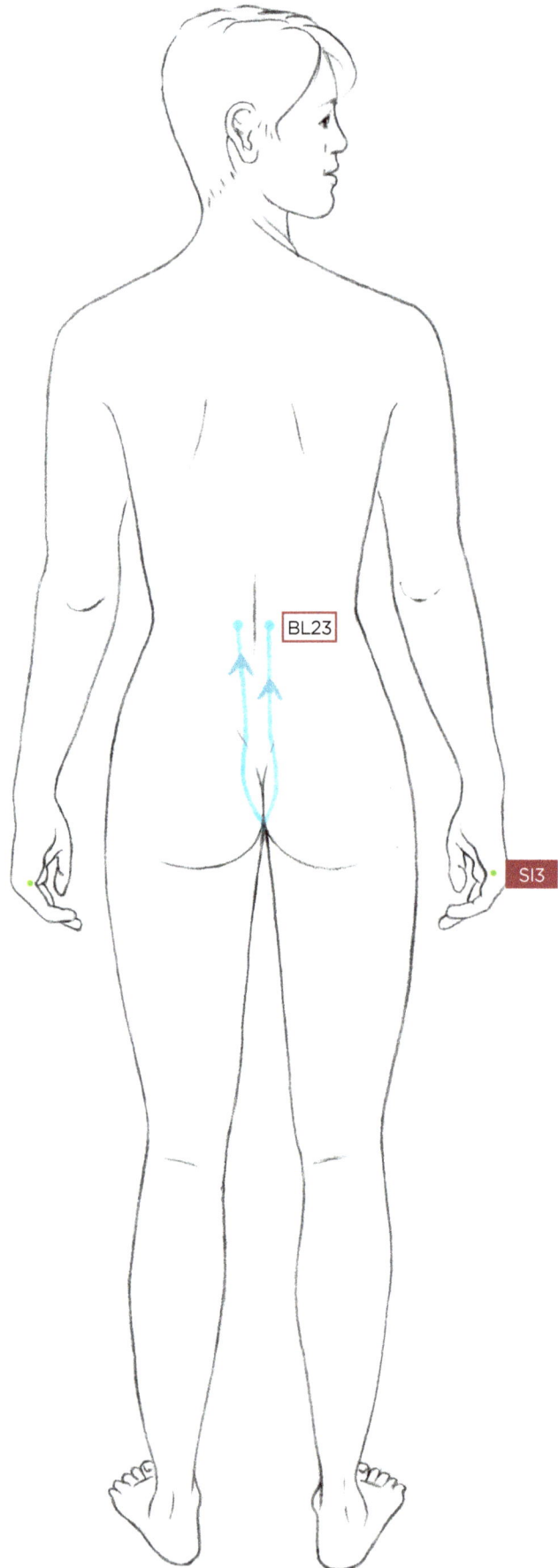

Du Mai

Fourth Trajectory

GV1   CV1

BL23

SI3

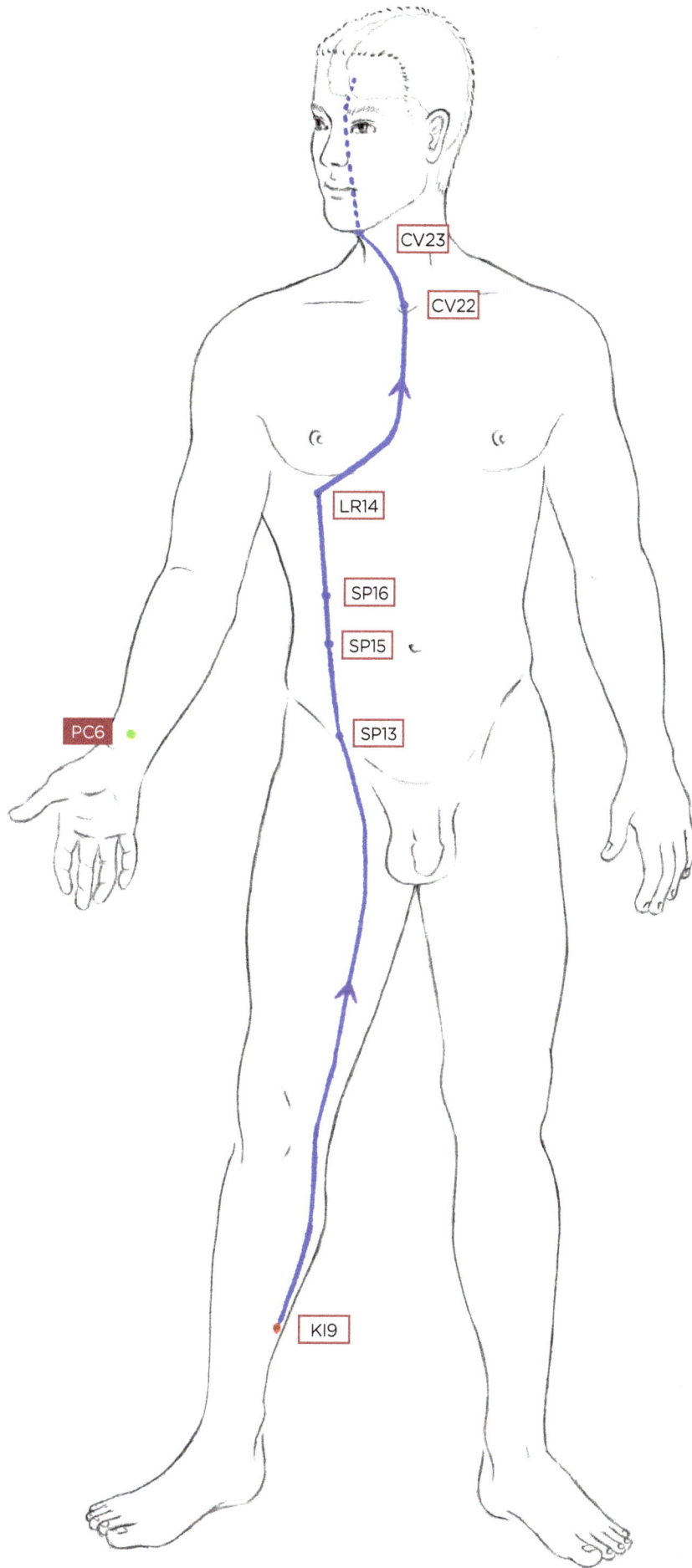

CV23

CV22

LR14

SP16

SP15

PC6

SP13

KI9

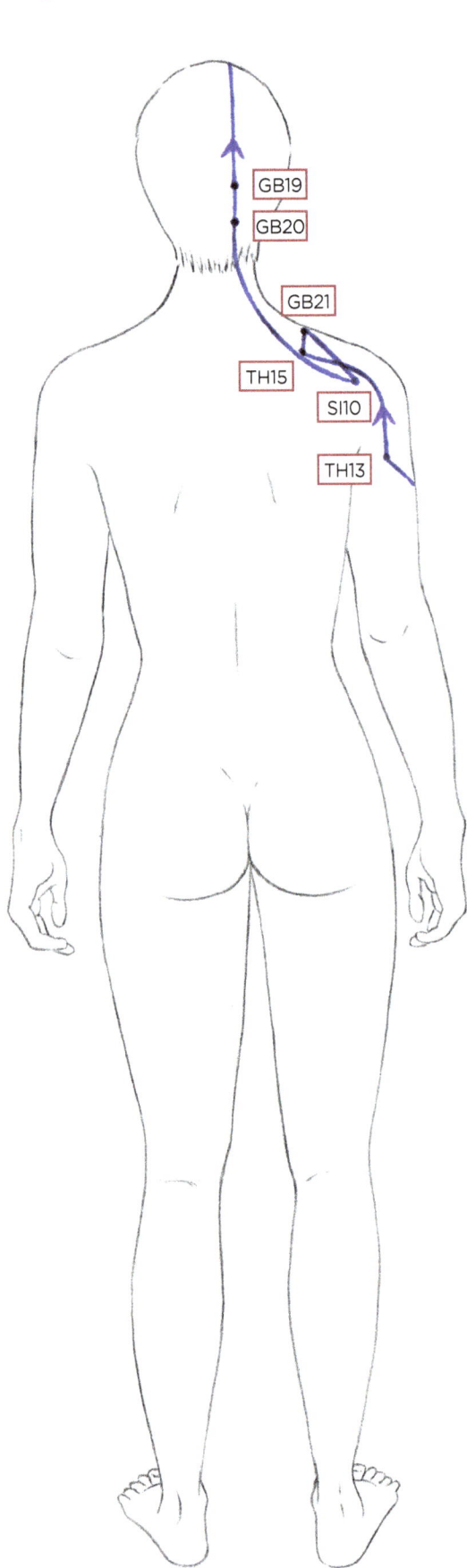

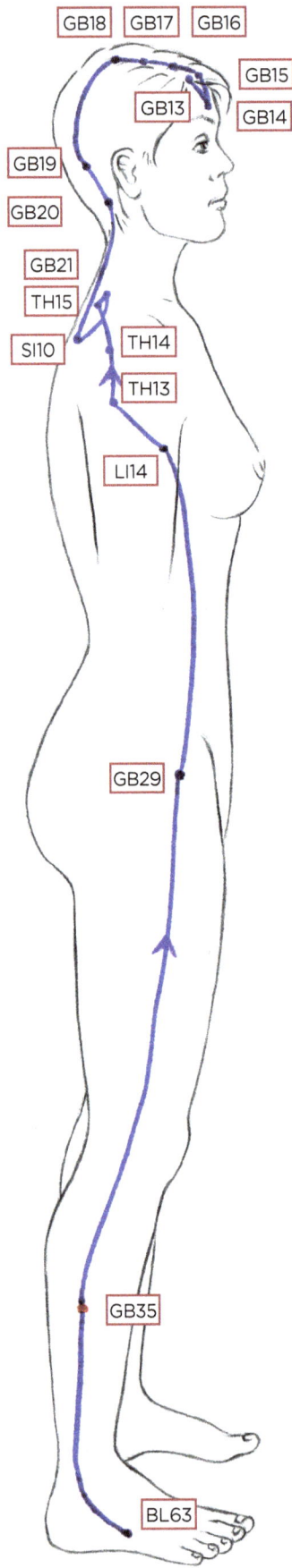

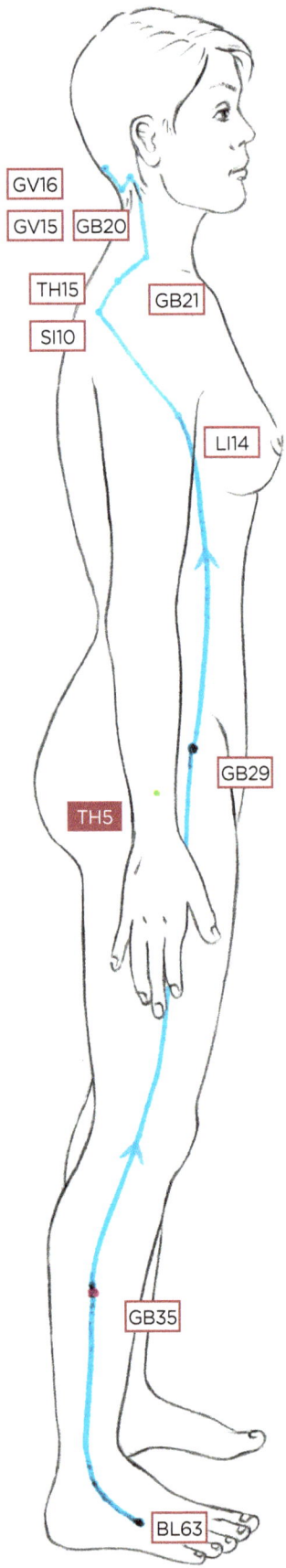

Yang Wei Mai

GB18   GB17   GB16
                GB15
        GB13   GB14

GB19
GB20

GB21
TH15
SI10   TH14
            TH13

        LI14

GB19
GB20

GB21

TH15

SI10

TH13

GV16
GV15   GB20

TH15   GB21
SI10

        LI14

GB29

TH5

GB29

GB35

GB35

BL63

BL63

Li Shi Zhen

Alternative

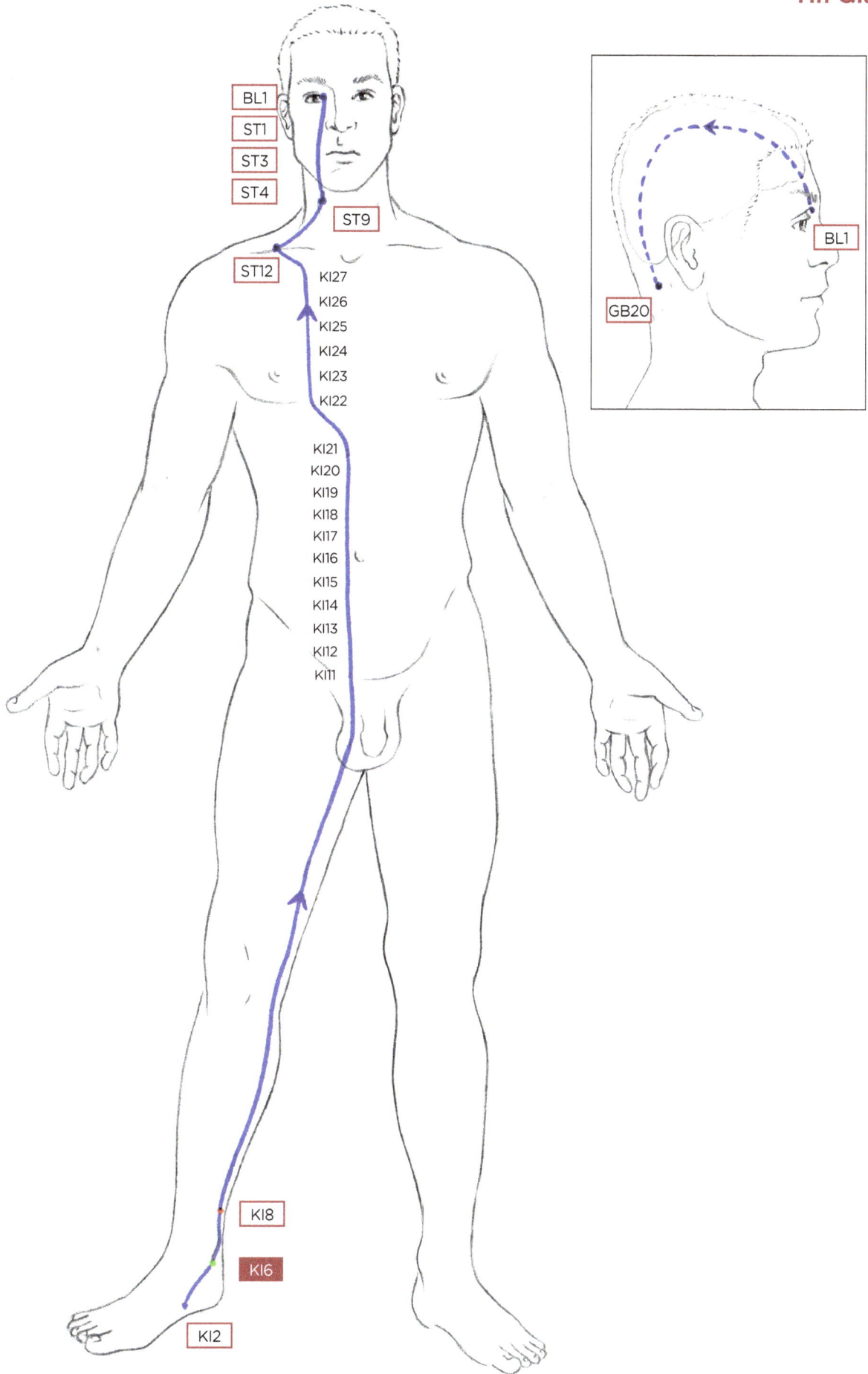

BL1
ST1
ST3
ST4
ST9
ST12

KI27
KI26
KI25
KI24
KI23
KI22

KI21
KI20
KI19
KI18
KI17
KI16
KI15
KI14
KI13
KI12
KI11

KI8
KI6
KI2

BL1
GB20

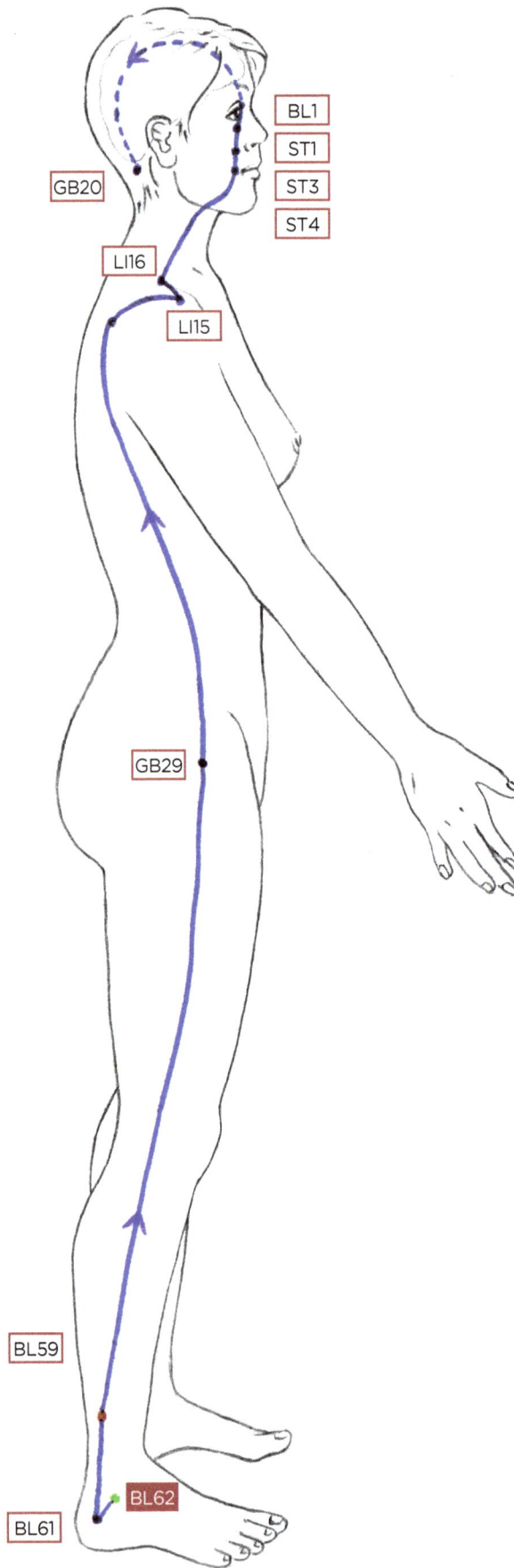

BL1

ST1

ST3

ST4

GB20

LI16

LI15

GB29

BL59

BL62

BL61

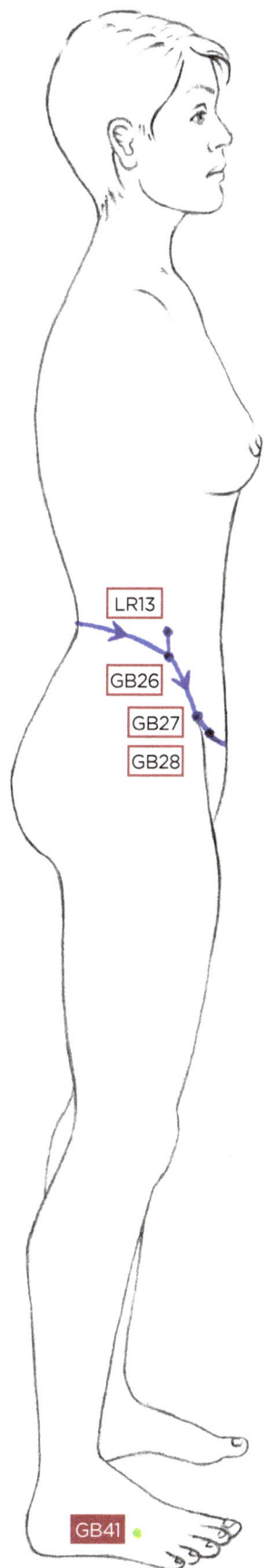

LR13

GB26

GB27

GB28

GB41

Draining Dai

GV4

BL23

BL52

GB26

SP15

ST25

KI16

CV8

GB41

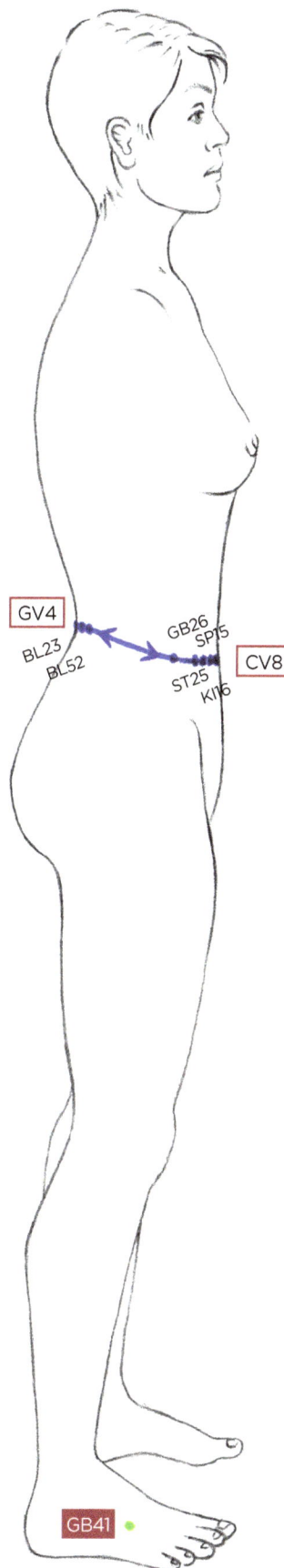

Consolidating Dai

Da Bao Mai

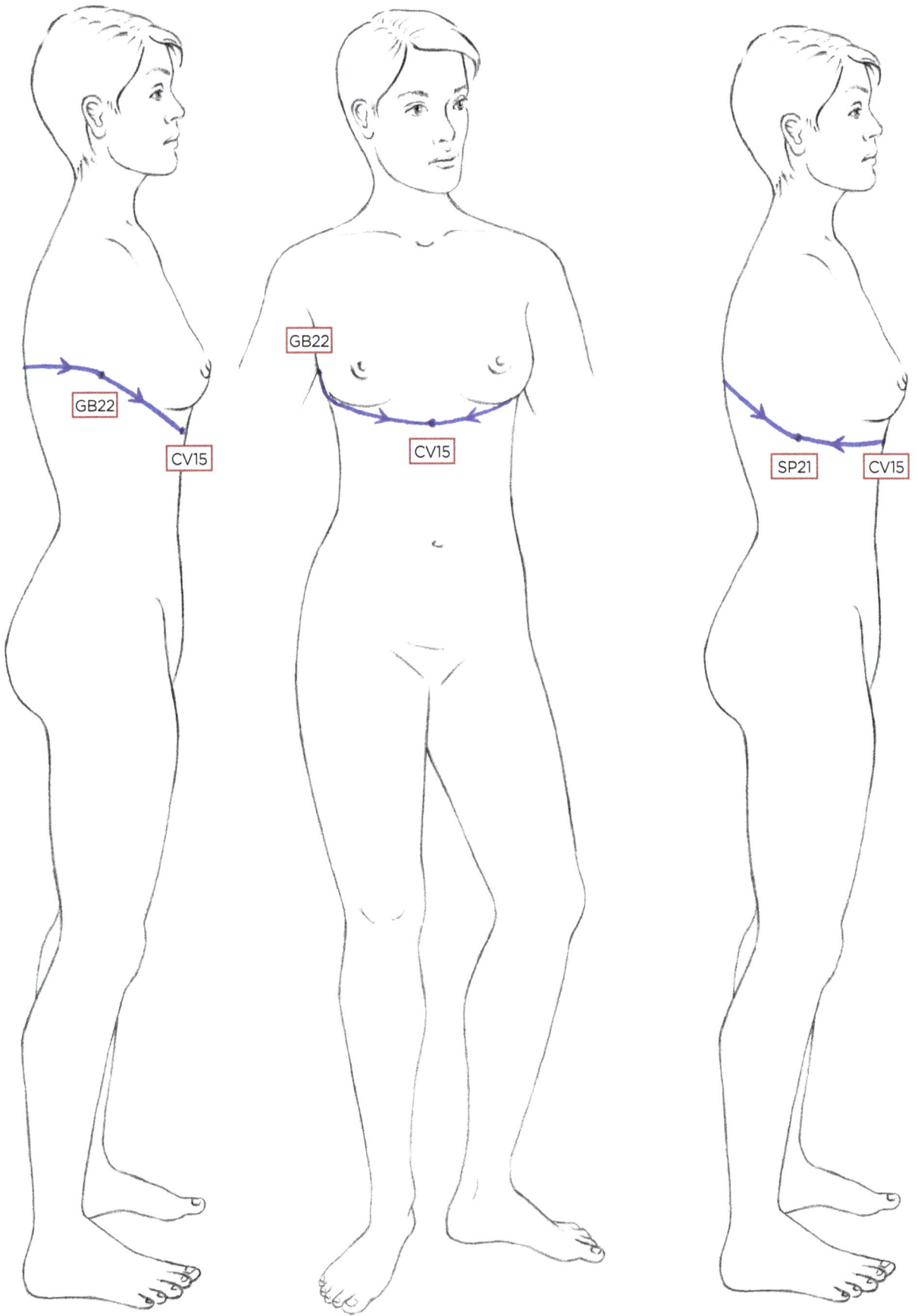

GB22

CV15

GB22

CV15

GB22

SP21   CV15

Draining Da Bao

Consolidating Da Bao

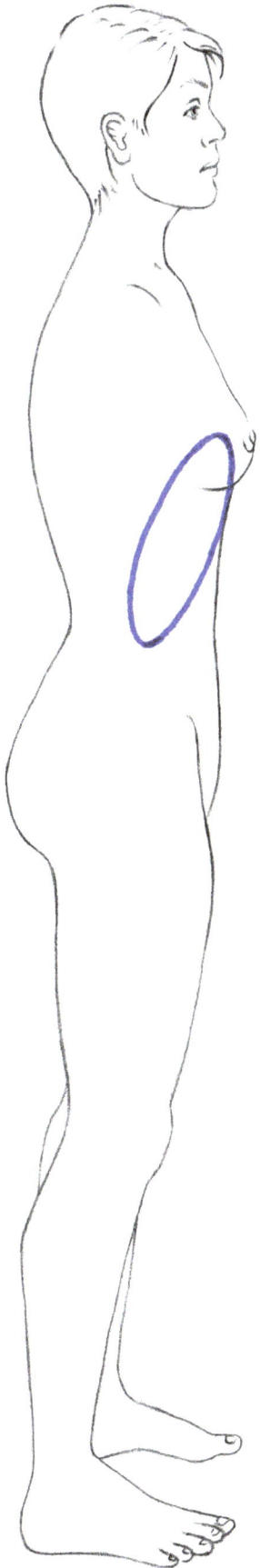

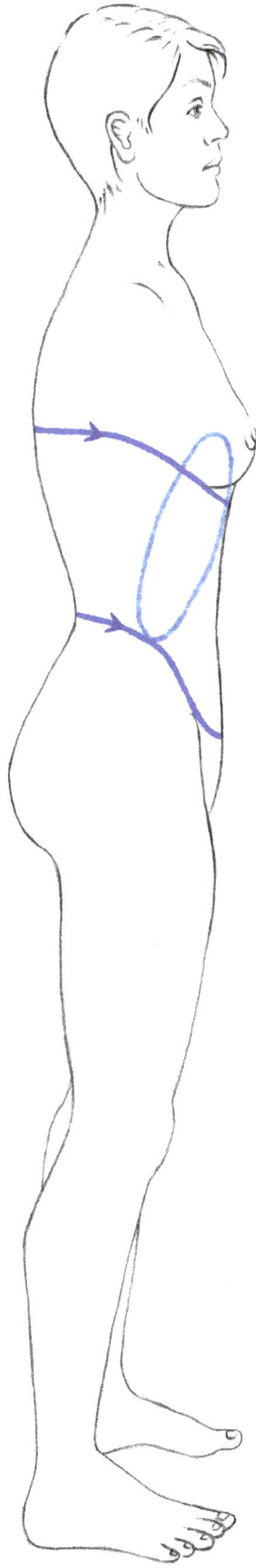

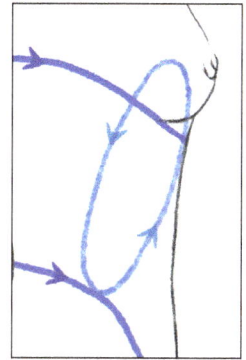

Women

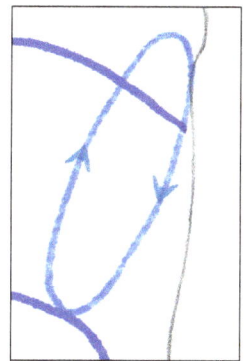

Men

8 EXTRA

Bao Mai

Bao Mai, Da Bao, Dai Mai

63

The Primary Channels

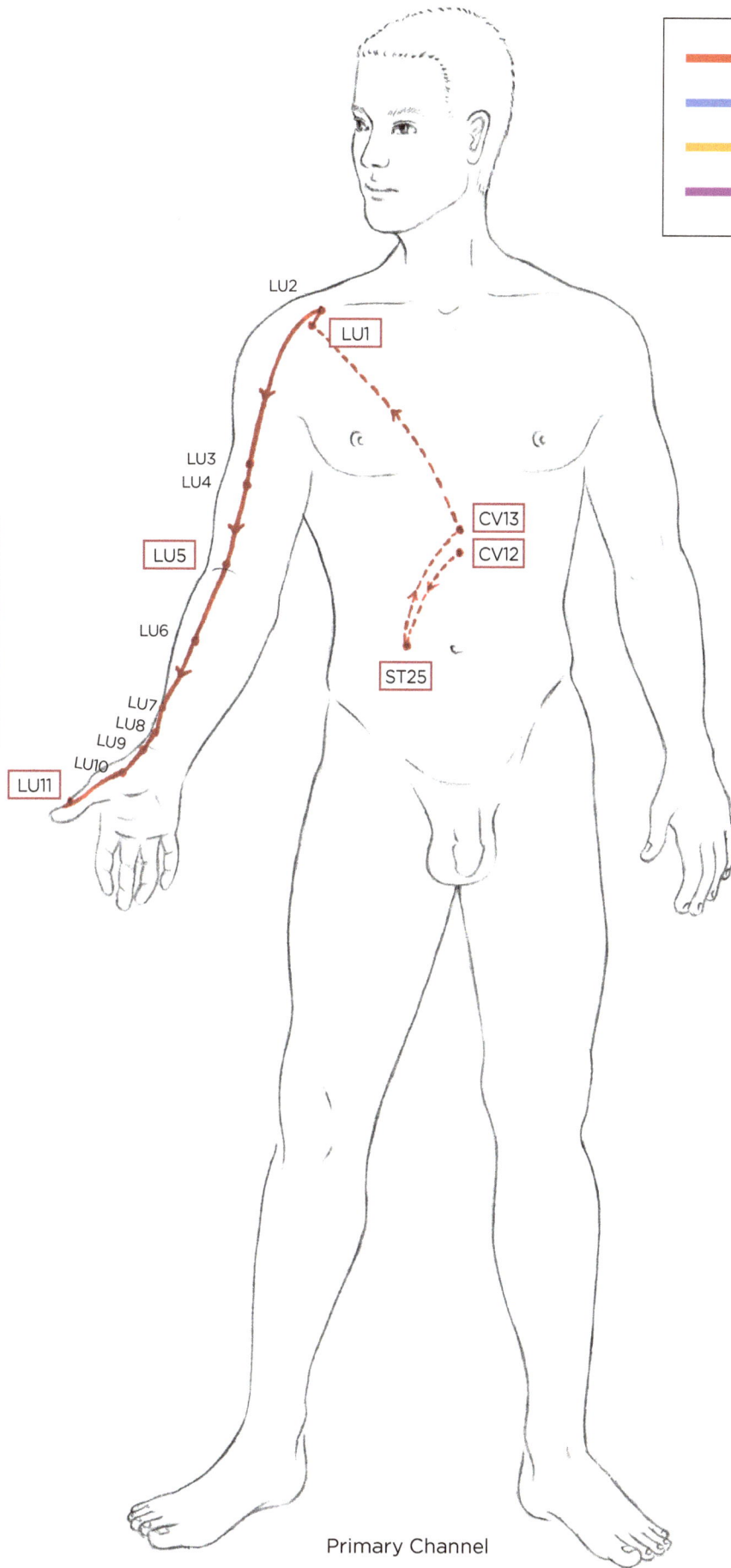

Primary Channel

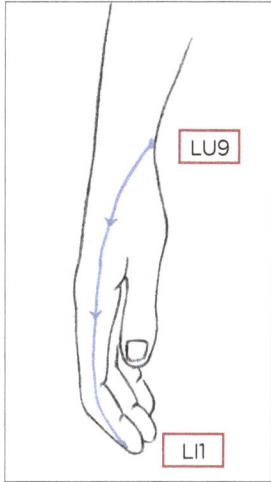

Branch 1

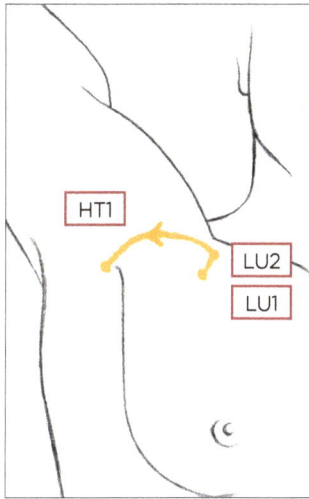

Branch 2

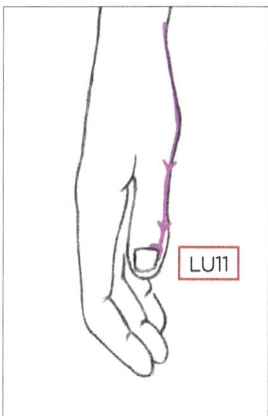

Branch 3

PRIMARY

Large Intestine Primary Channel

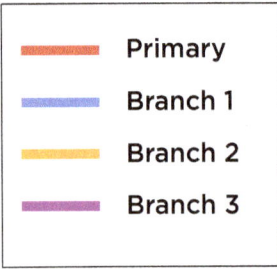

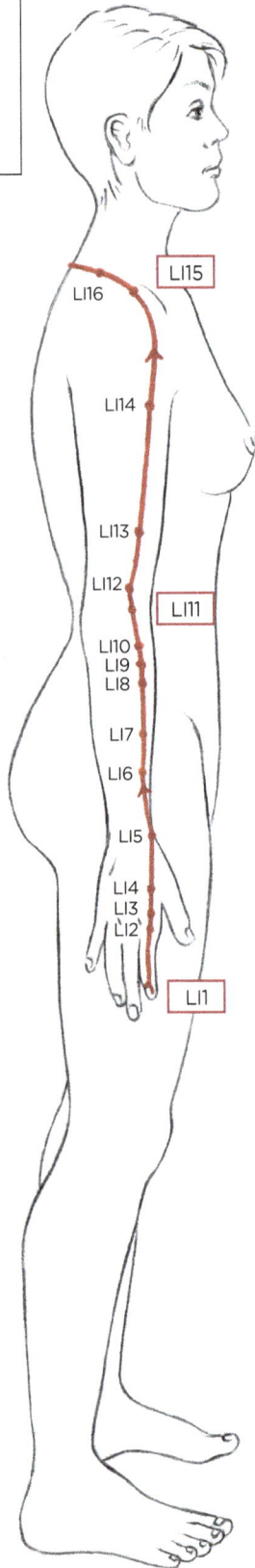

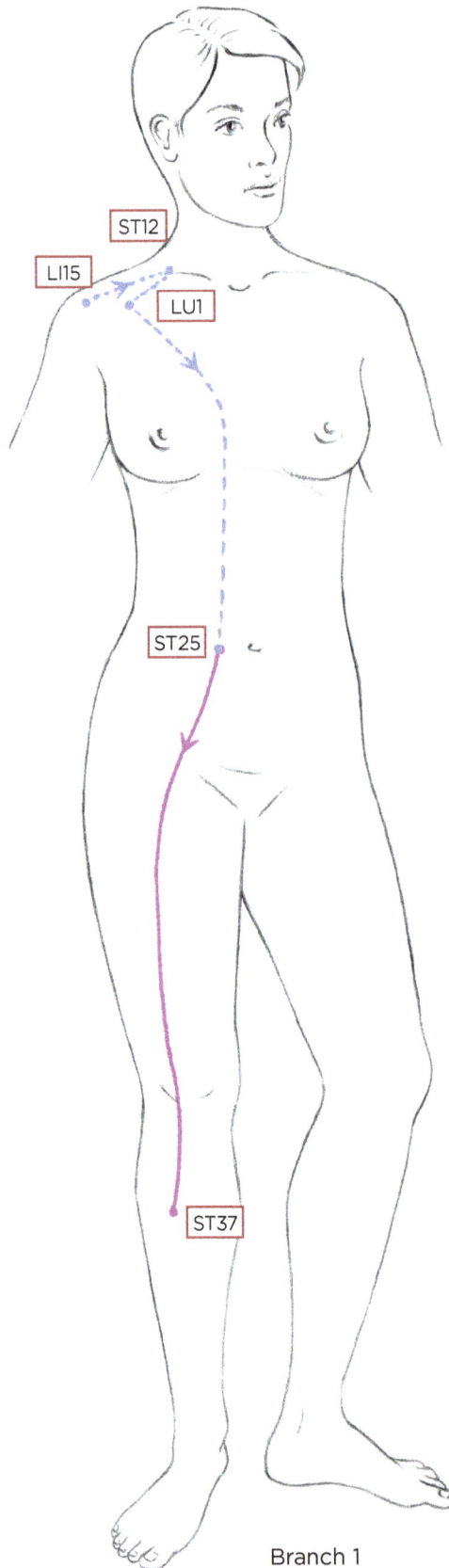

Legend:
- Primary
- Branch 1
- Branch 2
- Branch 3

Primary Channel (left figure, side view):
- LI16
- LI15
- LI14
- LI13
- LI12
- LI11
- LI10
- LI9
- LI8
- LI7
- LI6
- LI5
- LI4
- LI3
- LI2
- LI1

Primary Channel

Branch 1 / Branch 3 (center figure):
- ST12
- LI15
- LU1
- ST25
- ST37

Branch 1
Branch 3

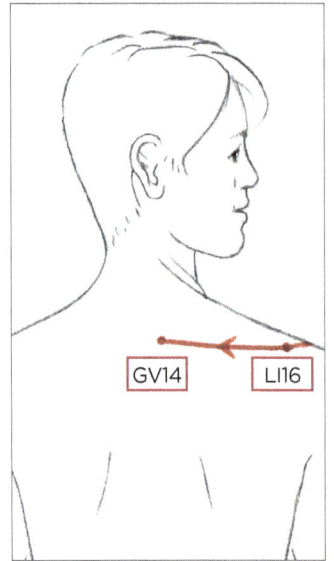

Primary - detail (upper right):
- GV14
- LI16

Primary - detail

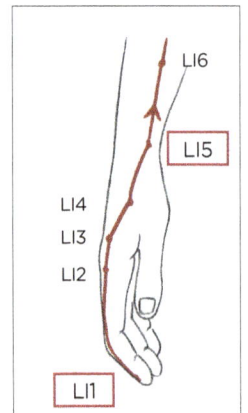

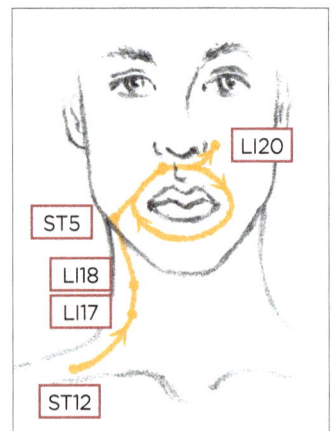

Primary - detail (middle right, arm/hand):
- LI6
- LI5
- LI4
- LI3
- LI2
- LI1

Primary - detail

Branch 2 (lower right, face):
- LI20
- ST5
- LI18
- LI17
- ST12

Branch 2

PRIMARY

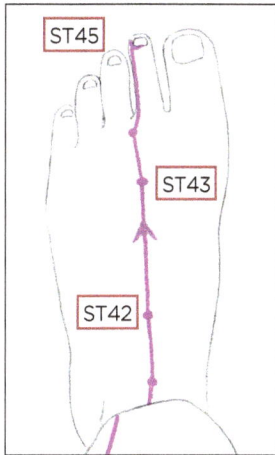

Branch 3 - detail

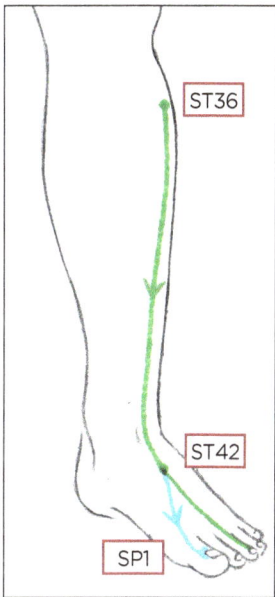

ST45
ST43
ST42

ST36
ST42
SP1

Branch 4
Branch 5

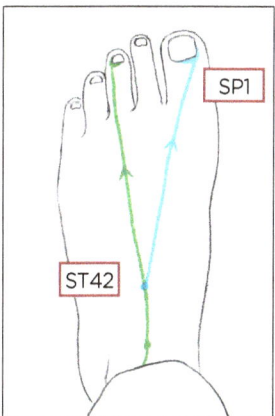

Branch 4 - detail
Branch 5

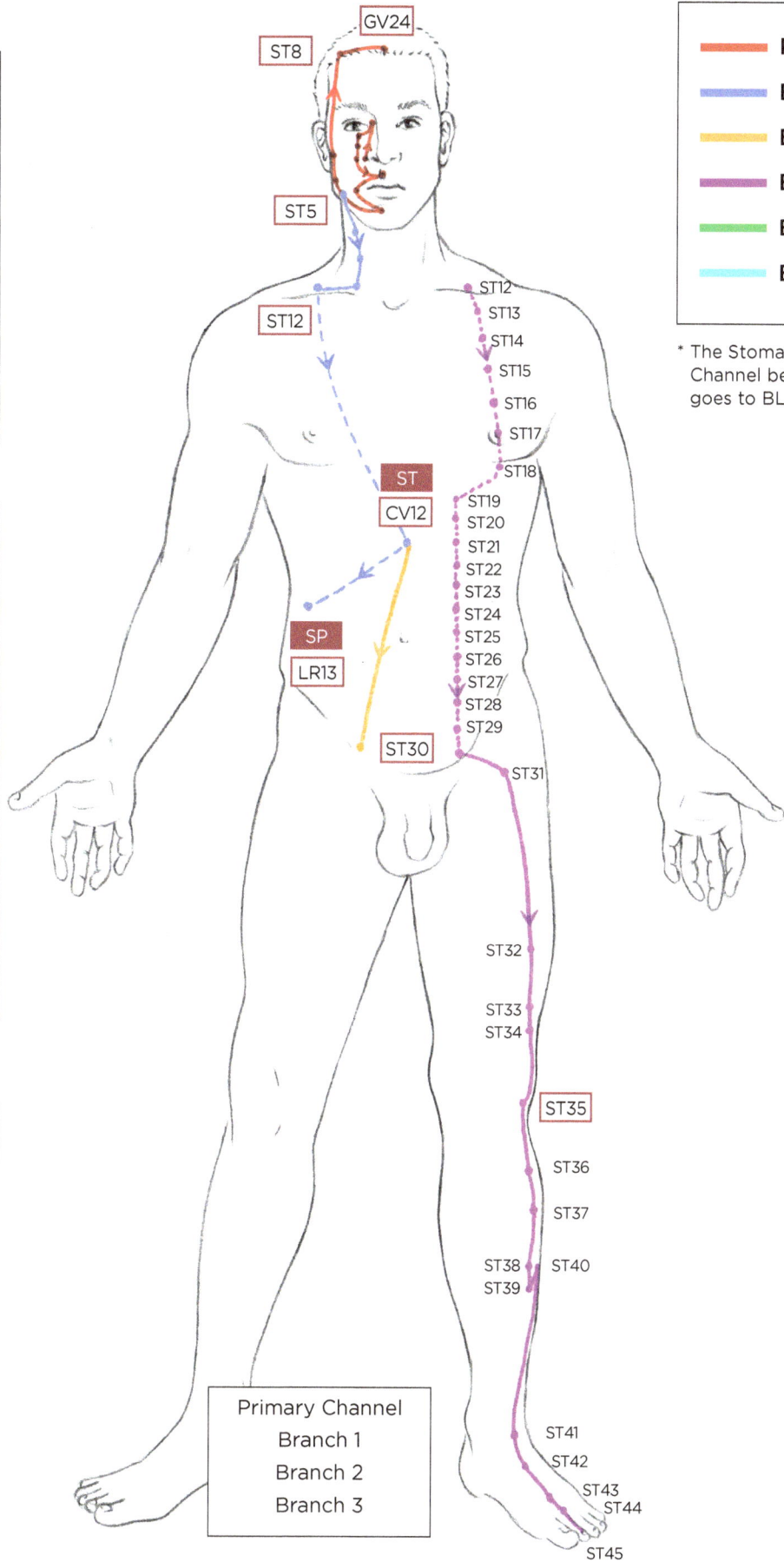

SP1
ST42

GV24
ST8
ST5
ST12
ST12
ST
CV12
SP
LR13
ST30

ST12
ST13
ST14
ST15
ST16
ST17
ST18
ST19
ST20
ST21
ST22
ST23
ST24
ST25
ST26
ST27
ST28
ST29
ST31
ST32
ST33
ST34
ST35
ST36
ST37
ST38
ST39
ST40
ST41
ST42
ST43
ST44
ST45

	Primary
	Branch 1
	Branch 2
	Branch 3
	Branch 4
	Branch 5

* The Stomach Primary
Channel begins at LI-20,
goes to BL-1, then ST-1.

PRIMARY

Primary Channel
Branch 1
Branch 2
Branch 3

Spleen Primary Channel

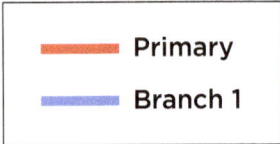

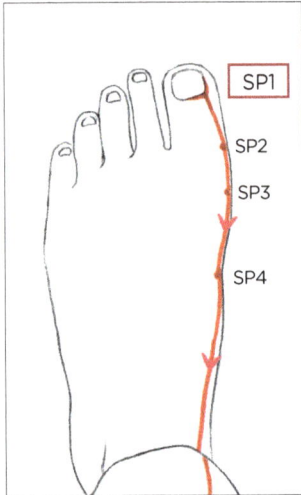

Legend:
- Primary
- Branch 1

Primary - detail

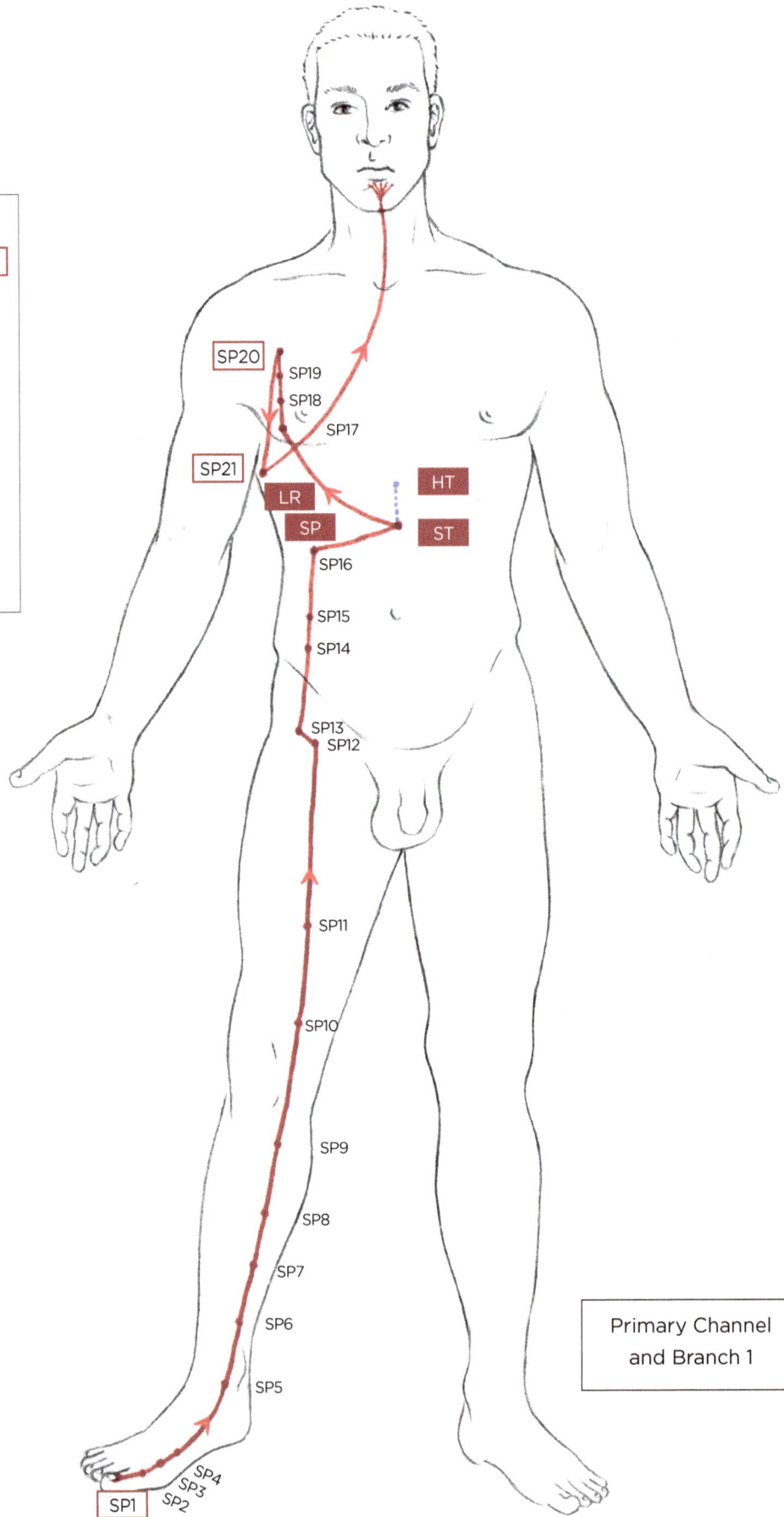

SP1
SP2
SP3
SP4

PRIMARY

SP20
SP19
SP18
SP17
SP21
LR
HT
SP
ST
SP16
SP15
SP14
SP13
SP12
SP11
SP10
SP9
SP8
SP7
SP6
SP5
SP4
SP3
SP2
SP1

Primary Channel
and Branch 1

Heart Primary Channel

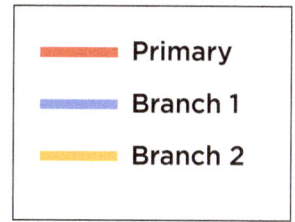

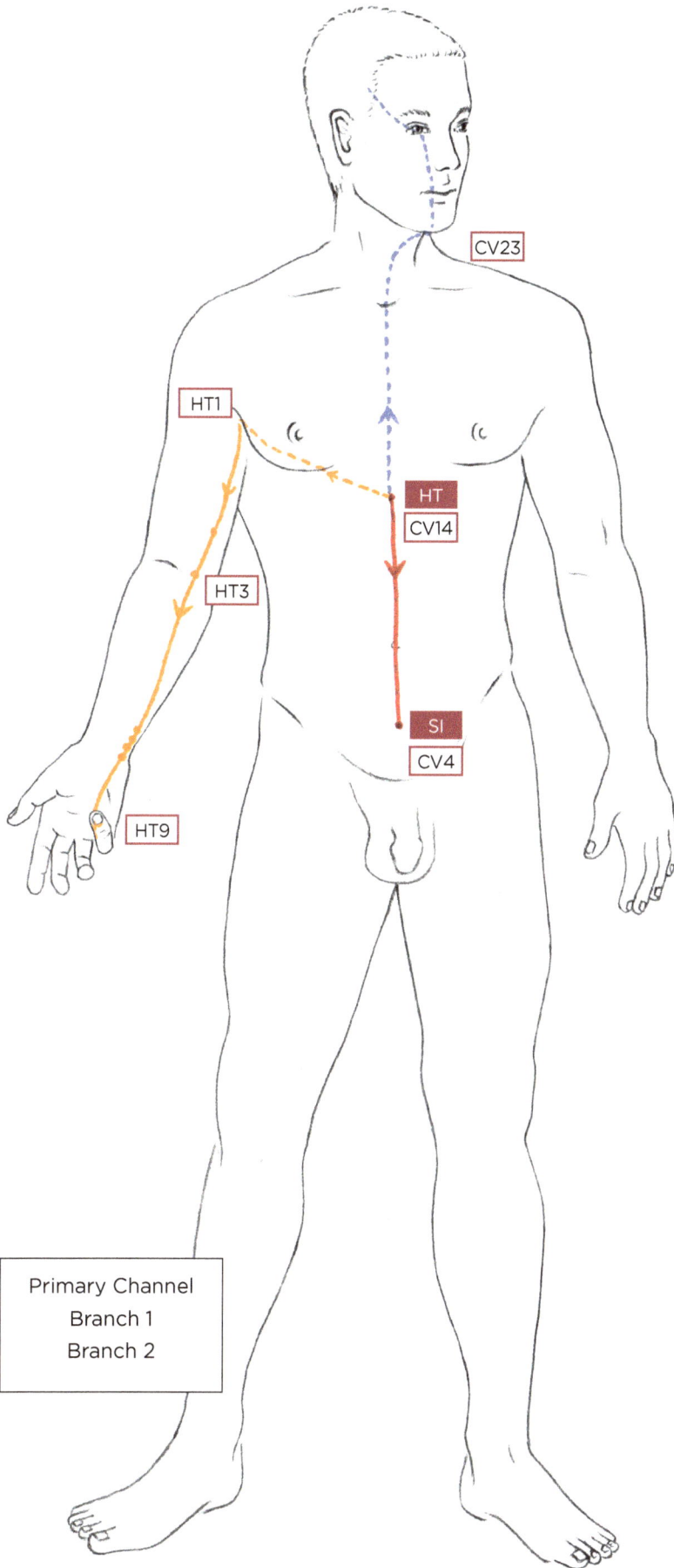

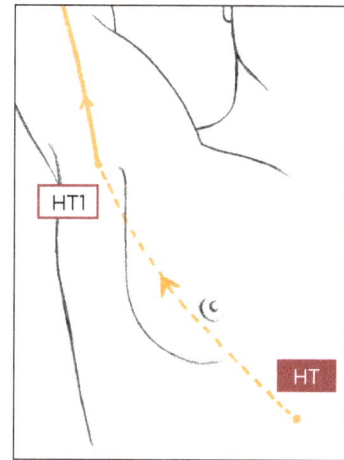

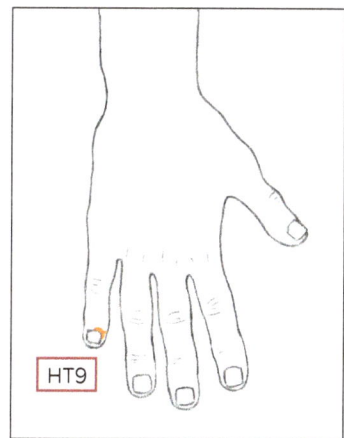

Primary
Branch 1
Branch 2

CV23

HT1

HT

CV14

HT3

SI

CV4

HT9

Branch 2 - detail

HT1

HT

Branch 2 - detail

HT9

PRIMARY

Primary Channel
Branch 1
Branch 2

69

Small Intestine Primary Channel

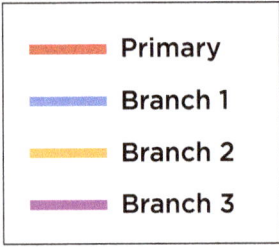

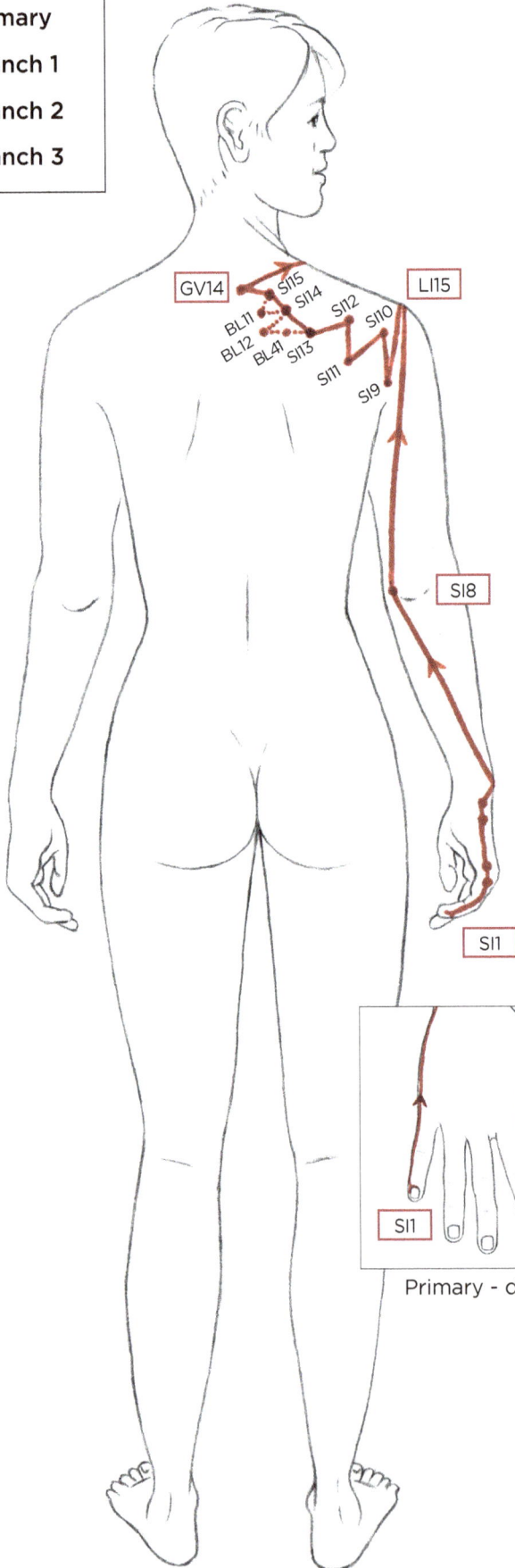

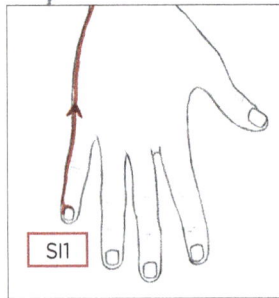

PRIMARY

Primary	
Branch 1	
Branch 2	
Branch 3	

GV14
SI15
SI14
BL11
SI12
BL12
BL41 SI13
SI11
SI10
SI9
LI15

SI8

SI1

SI19
BL1
SI18
SI16
ST12

CV14
CV13
CV12

CV4

ST39

SI1

Primary - detail

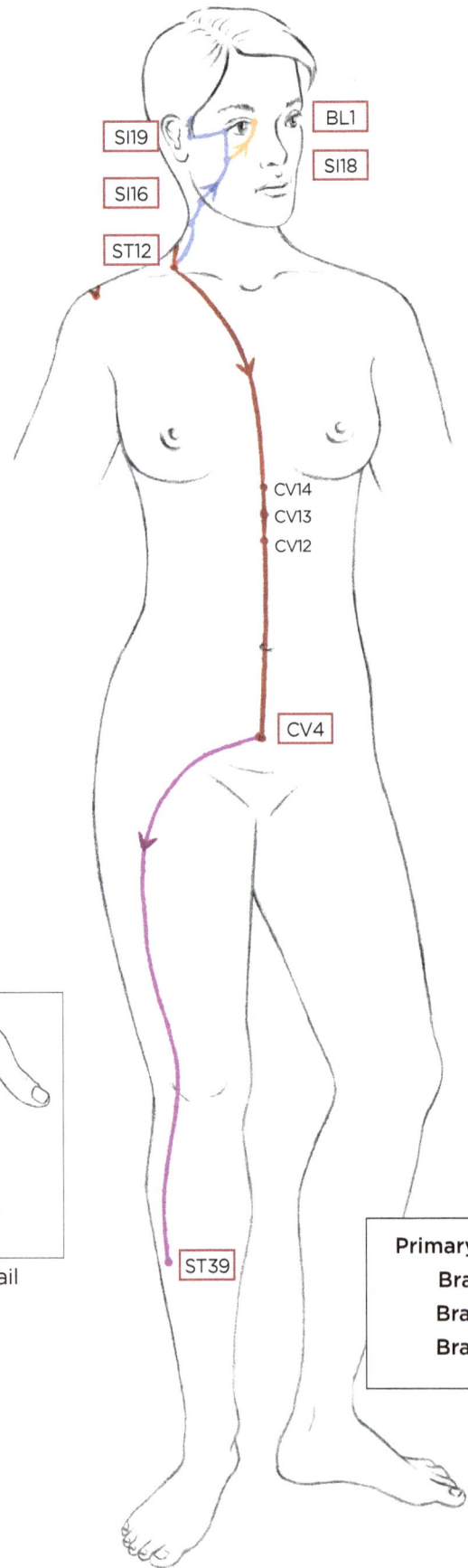

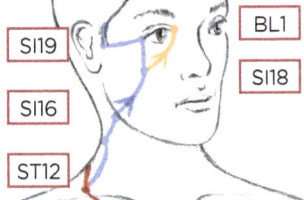

Primary Channel
Branch 1
Branch 2
Branch 3

Primary Channel

70

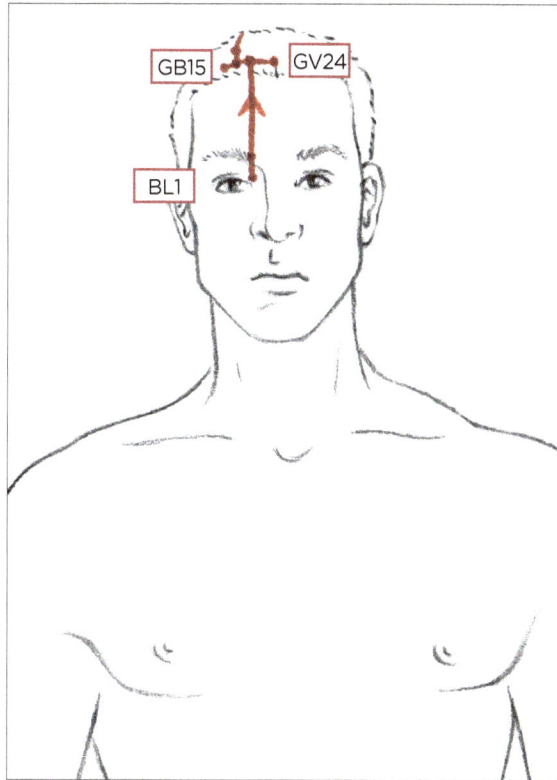

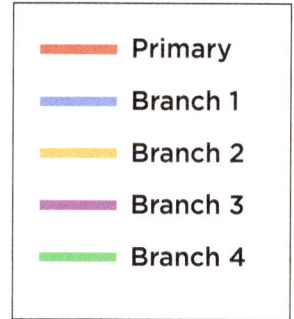

Primary Channel

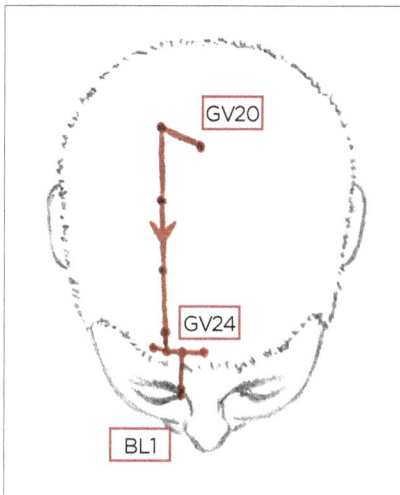

	Primary
	Branch 1
	Branch 2
	Branch 3
	Branch 4

Primary - detail

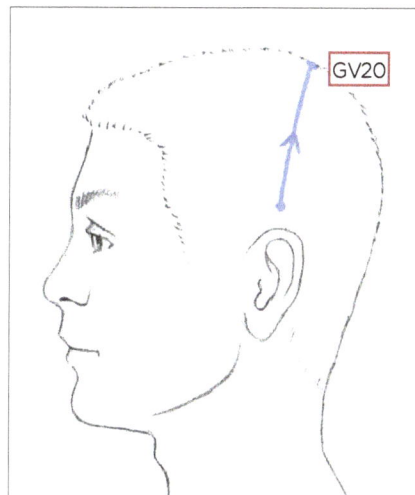

Branch 1

Bladder Primary Channel

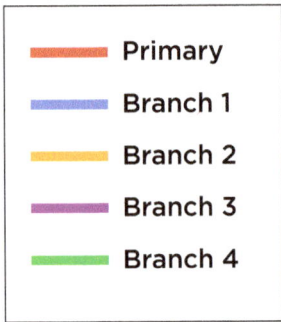

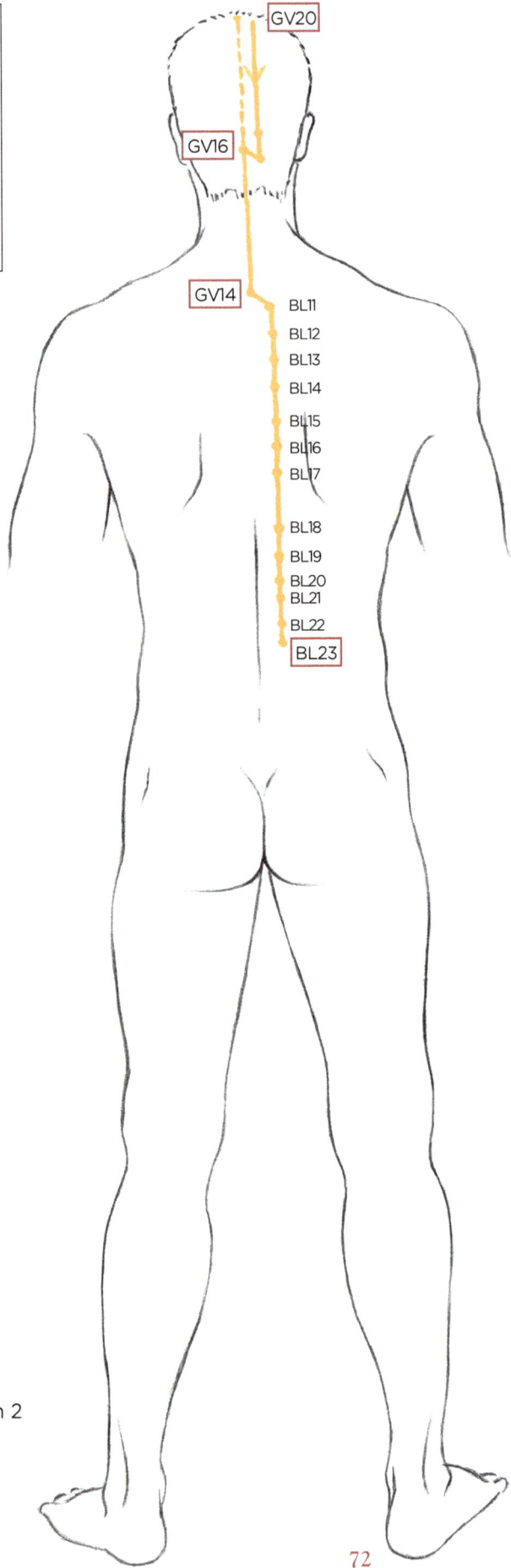

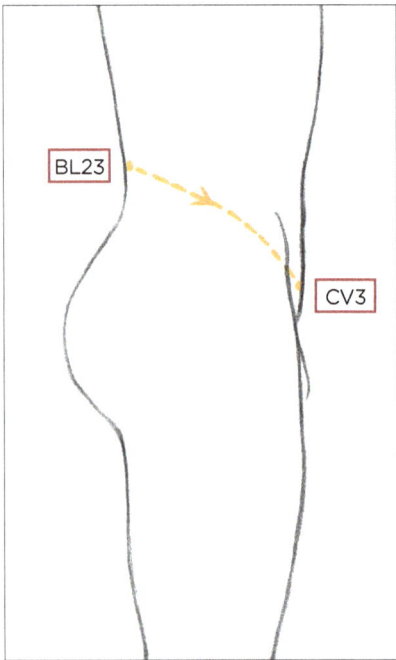

Primary	
Branch 1	
Branch 2	
Branch 3	
Branch 4	

PRIMARY

GV20

GV16

GV14

BL11
BL12
BL13
BL14
BL15
BL16
BL17
BL18
BL19
BL20
BL21
BL22
BL23

BL23

CV3

Branch 2 - detail

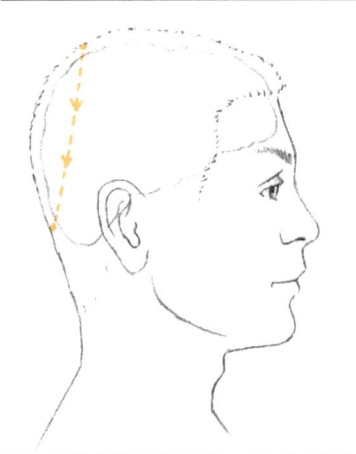

Branch 2 - detail

Branch 2

Bladder Primary Channel

- Primary
- Branch 1
- Branch 2
- Branch 3
- Branch 4

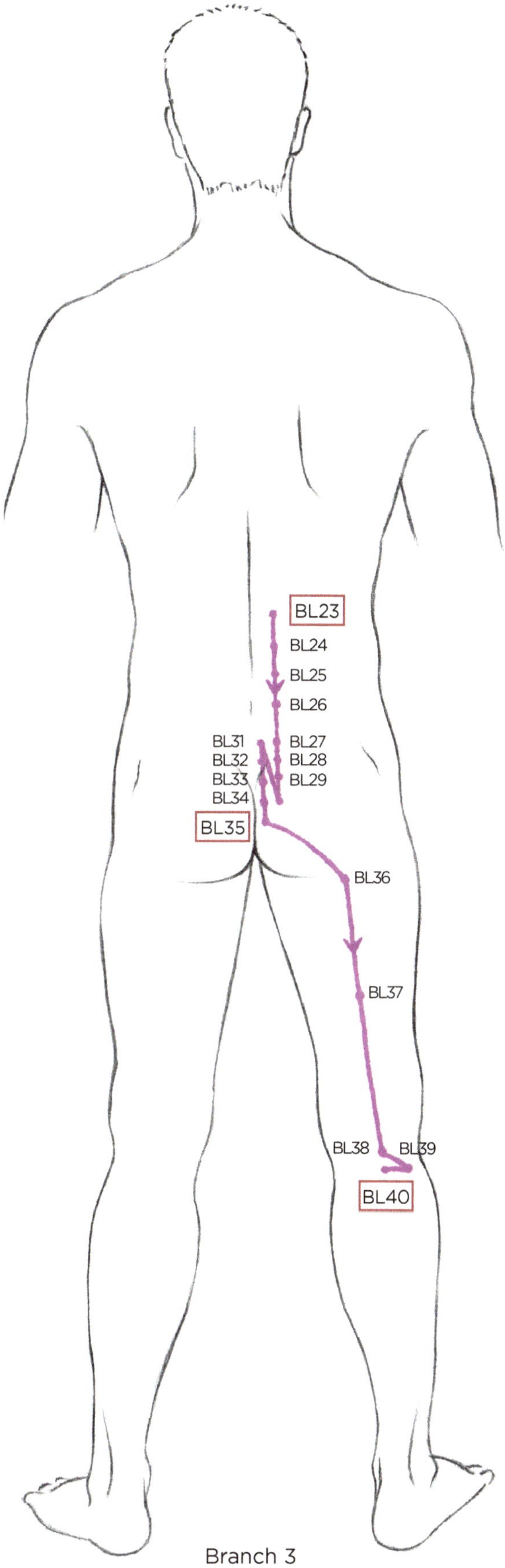
BL23
BL24
BL25
BL26
BL31
BL32
BL33
BL34
BL27
BL28
BL29
BL35
BL36
BL37
BL38
BL39
BL40

Branch 3

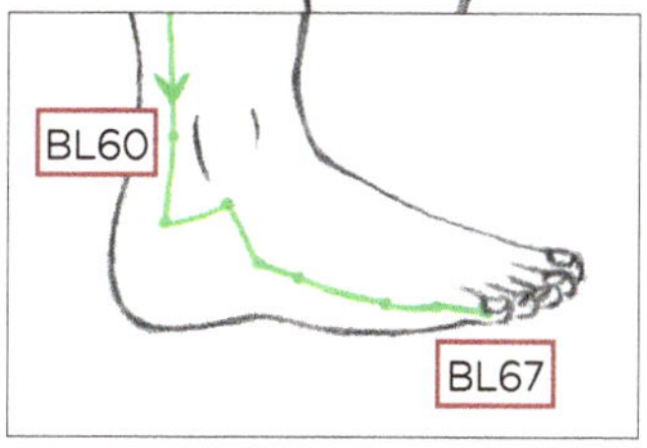
BL60
BL67

Branch 4 - detail

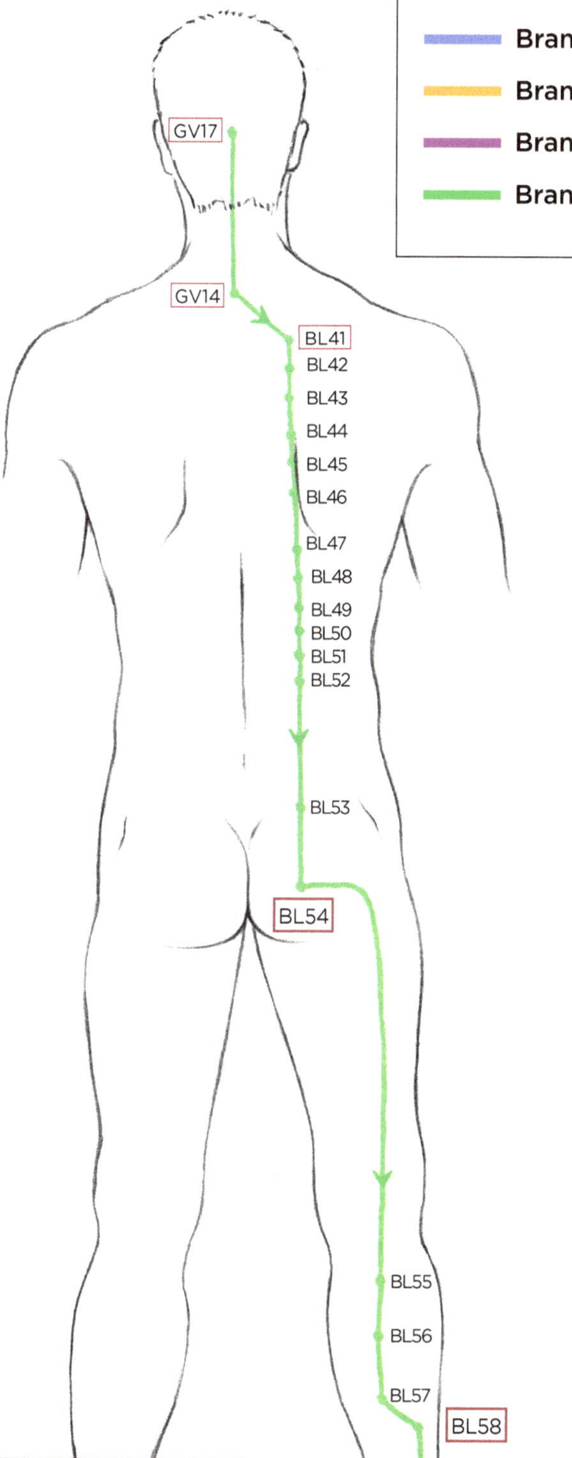
GV17
GV14
BL41
BL42
BL43
BL44
BL45
BL46
BL47
BL48
BL49
BL50
BL51
BL52
BL53
BL54
BL55
BL56
BL57
BL58
BL59
BL60
BL61
BL67

Branch 4

Kidney Primary Channel

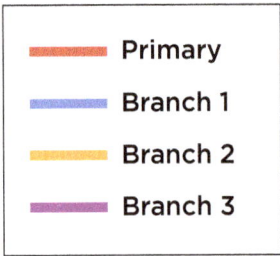

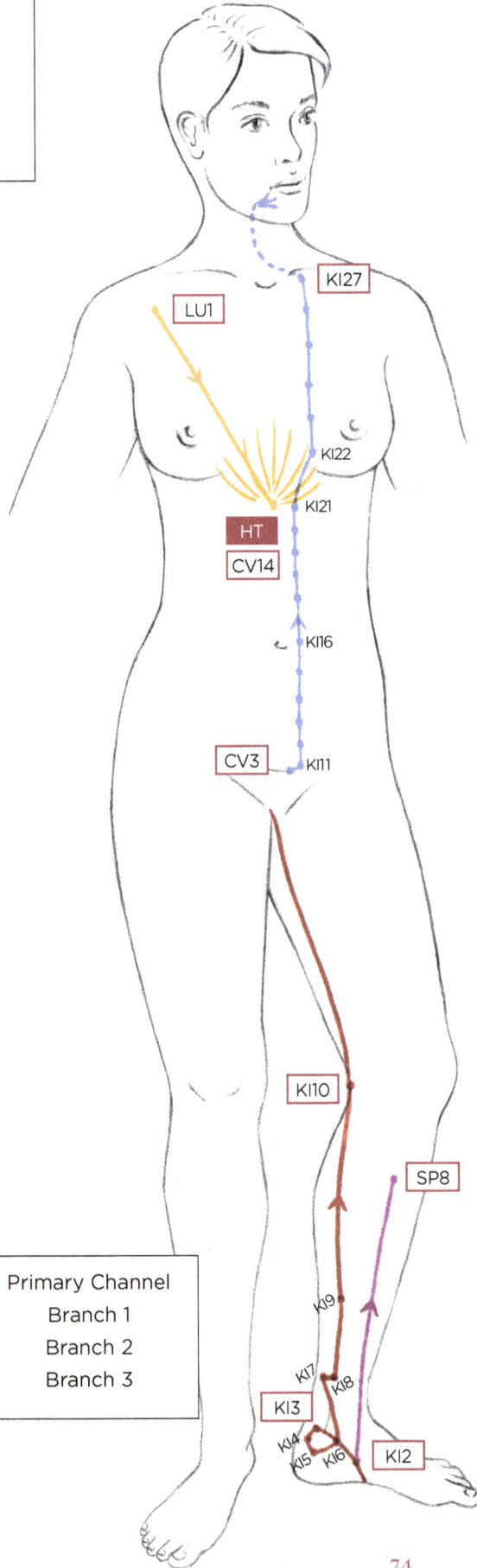

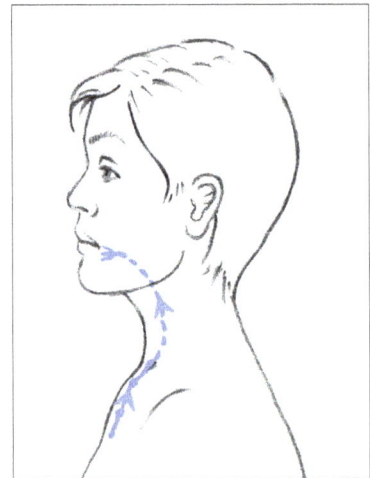

Primary
Branch 1
Branch 2
Branch 3

LU1

KI27

KI22

KI21

HT

CV14

KI16

CV3   KI11

KI10

SP8

KI9

KI7

KI3   KI8

KI4
KI5   KI6   KI2

PRIMARY

Primary Channel
Branch 1
Branch 2
Branch 3

Branch 1 - detail

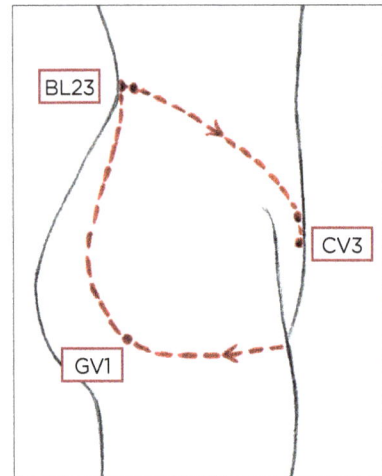

BL23

CV3

GV1

Primary - detail

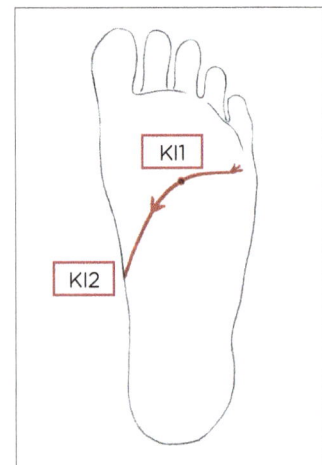

KI1

KI2

Primary - detail

74

	Primary
	Branch 1
	Branch 2

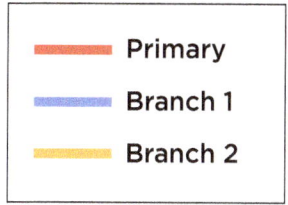

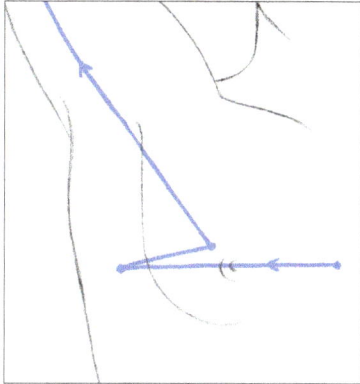

Branch 1 - detail

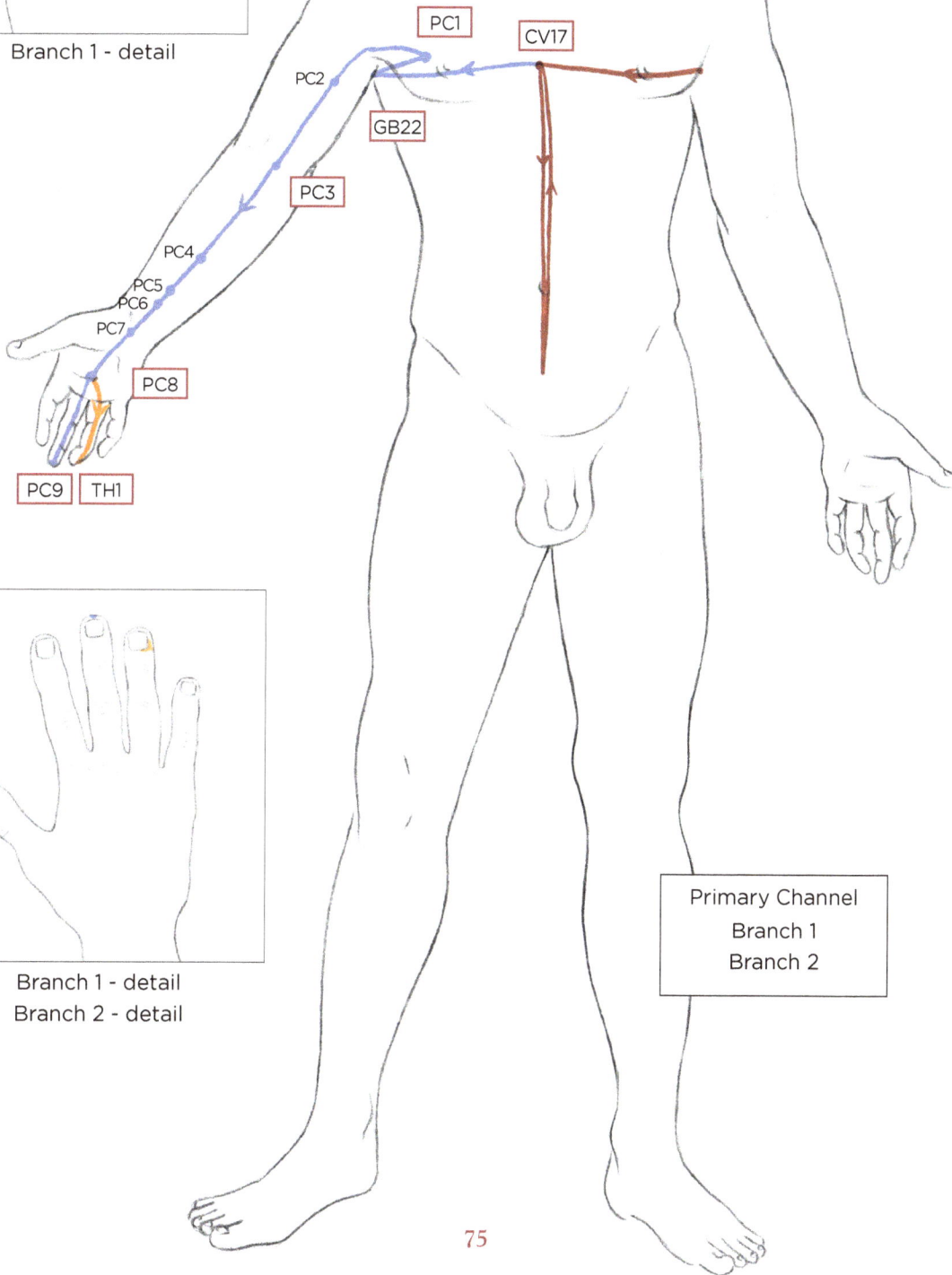

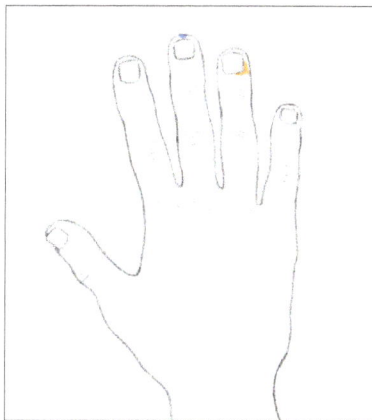

PC1

CV17

PC2

GB22

PC3

PC4

PC5

PC6

PC7

PC8

PC9   TH1

Branch 1 - detail
Branch 2 - detail

Primary Channel
Branch 1
Branch 2

PRIMARY

Triple Heater Primary Channel

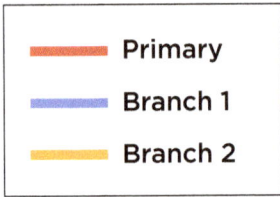

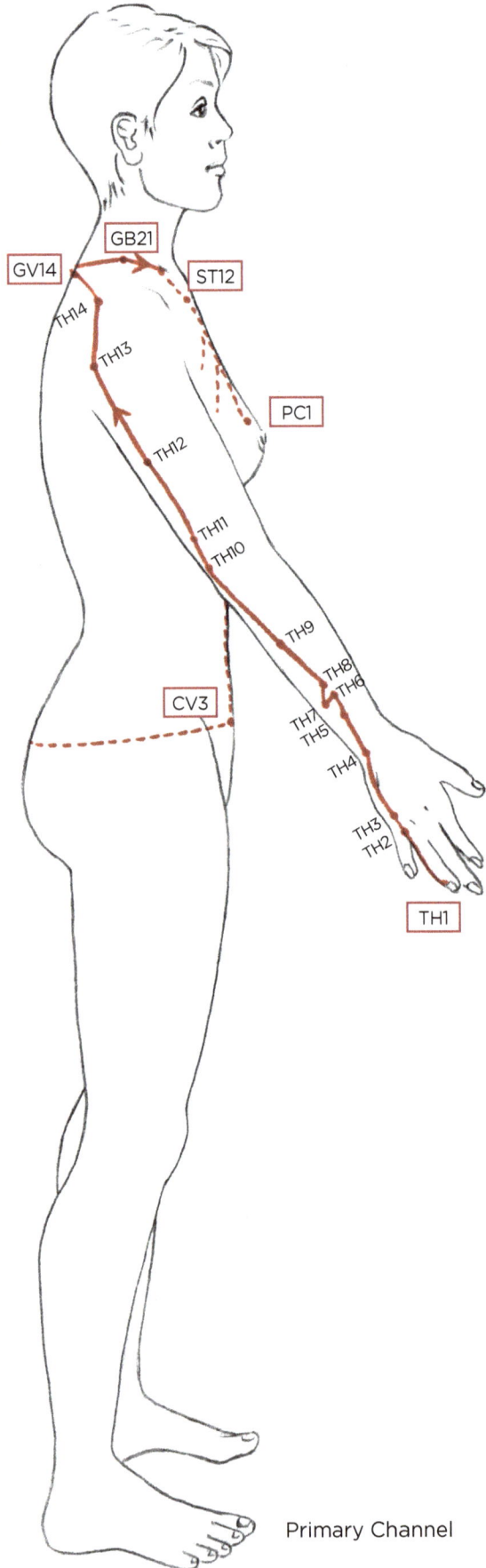

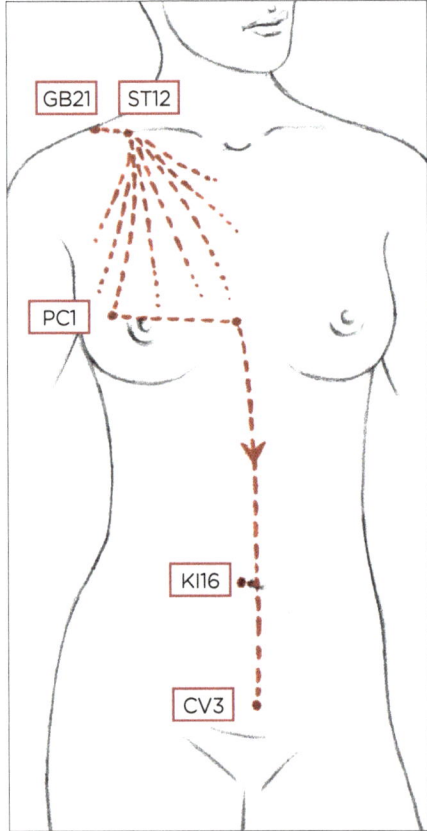

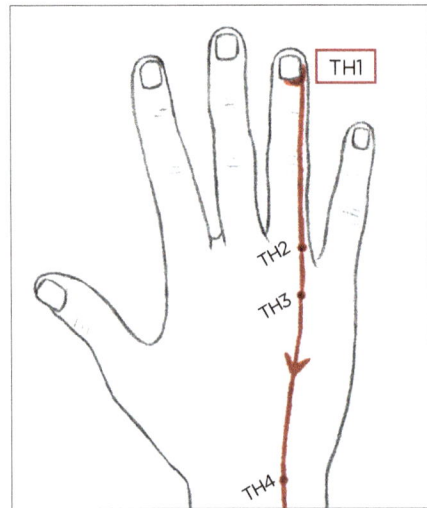

Legend:
- Primary
- Branch 1
- Branch 2

GV14

GB21

ST12

TH14

TH13

PC1

TH12

TH11
TH10

TH9

CV3

TH8
TH6

TH7
TH5

TH4

TH3
TH2

TH1

GB21 ST12

PC1

KI16

CV3

TH1

TH2

TH3

TH4

Primary Channel

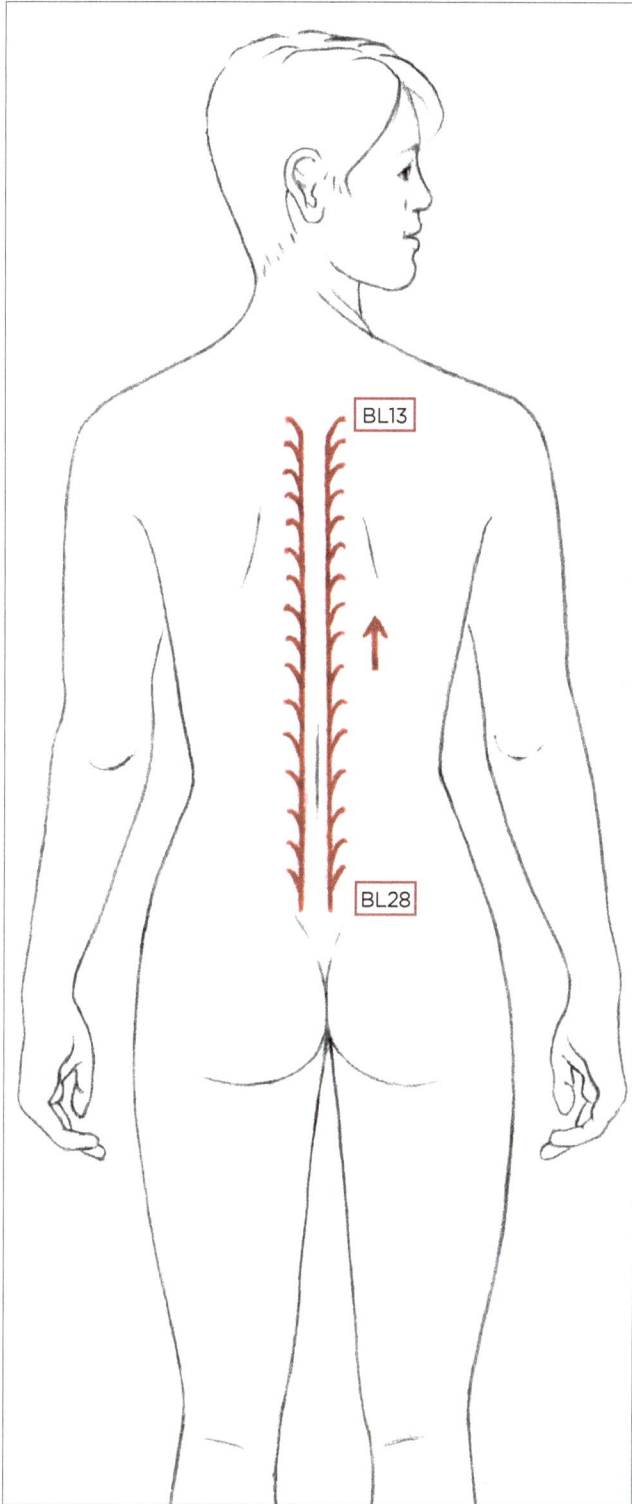

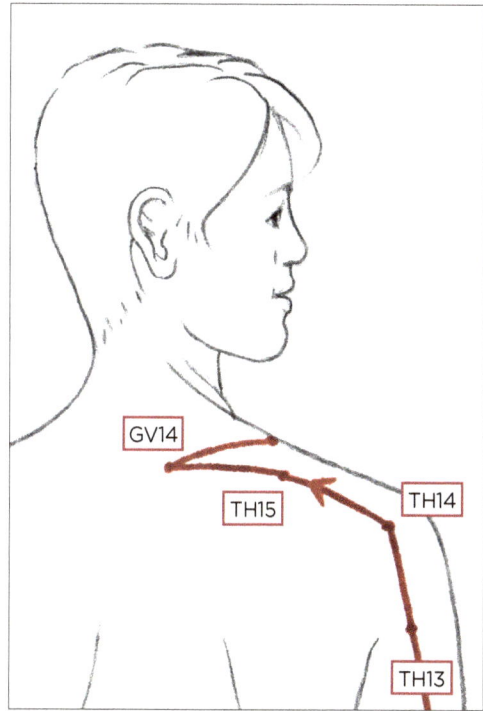

PRIMARY

Primary Channel

Triple Heater Primary Channel

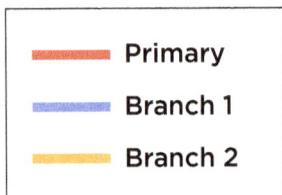

- Primary
- Branch 1
- Branch 2

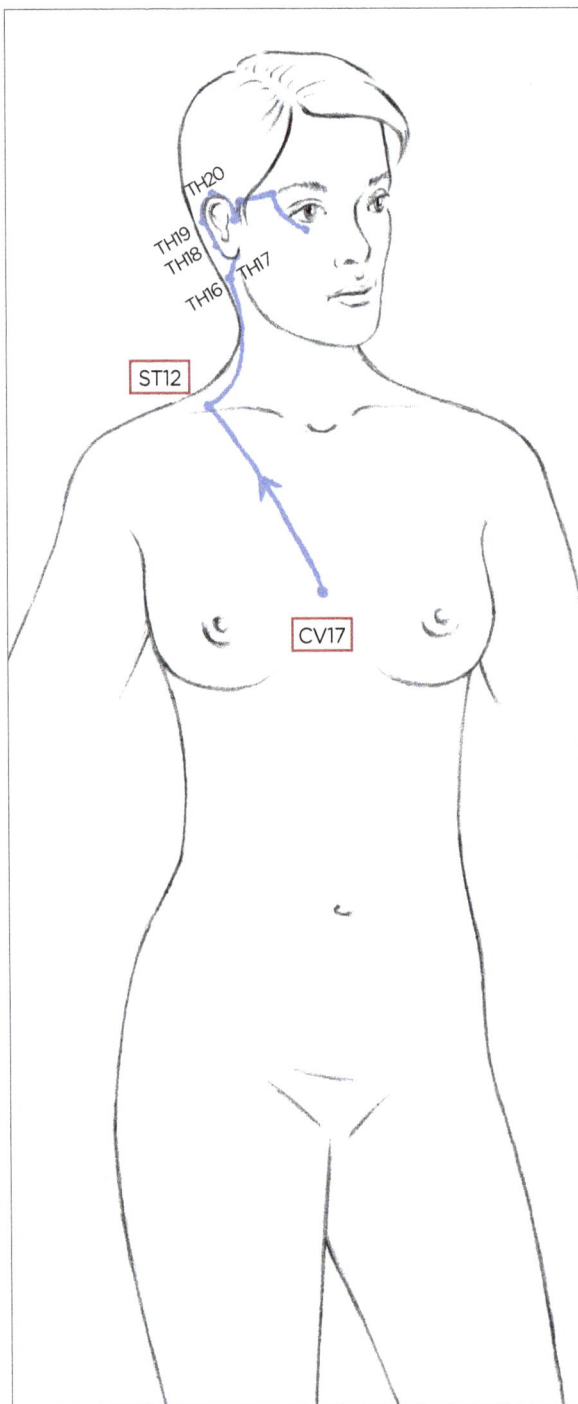

TH20
TH19
TH18
TH17
TH16
ST12
CV17

Branch 1

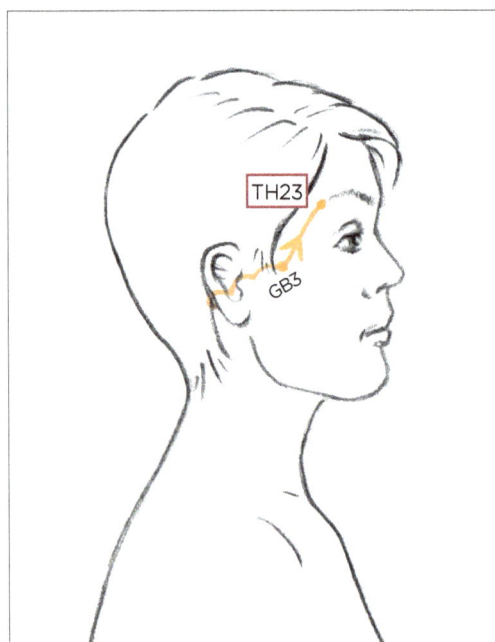

TH23
GB3

Branch 2

78

Primary
Branch 1
Branch 2
Branch 3
Branch 4

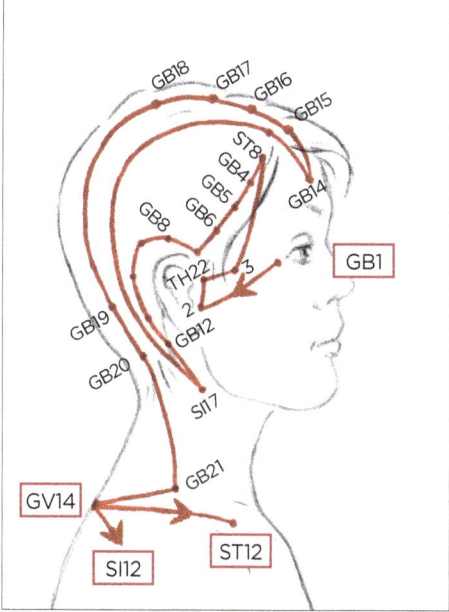

Primary Channel

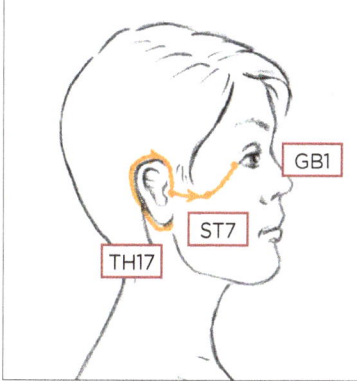

Branch 2

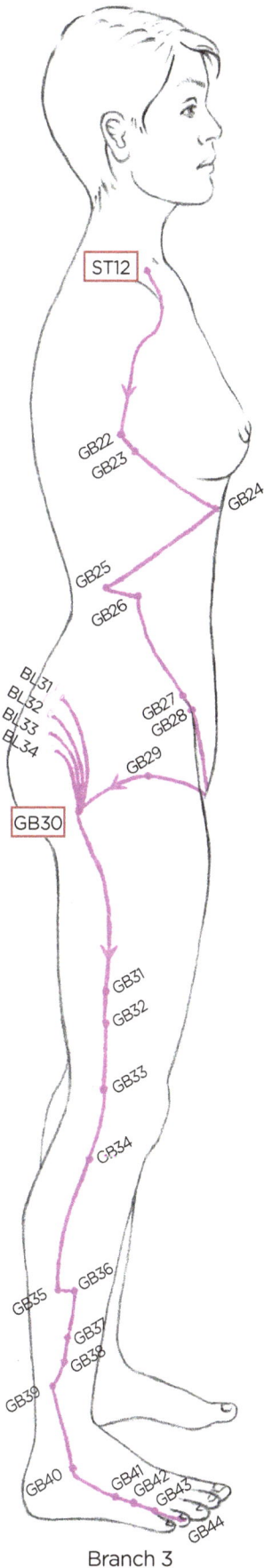

Branch 3

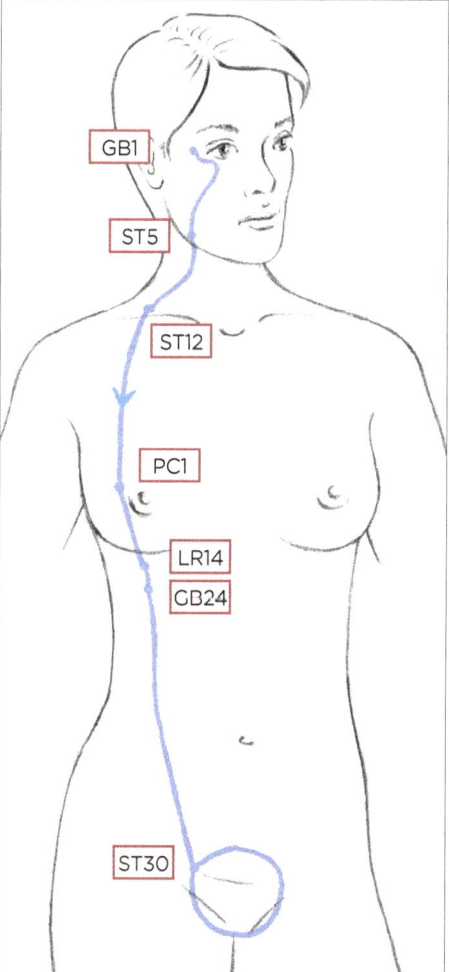

Branch 1

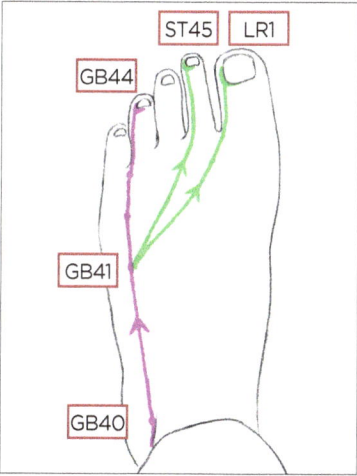

Branch 3 - detail
and Branch 4

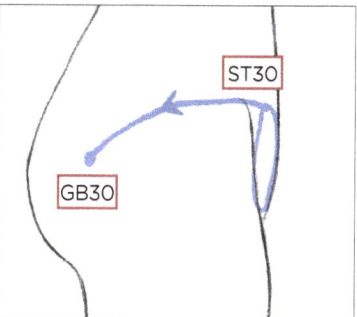

Branch 1 - detail

Liver Primary Channel

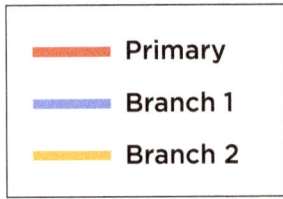

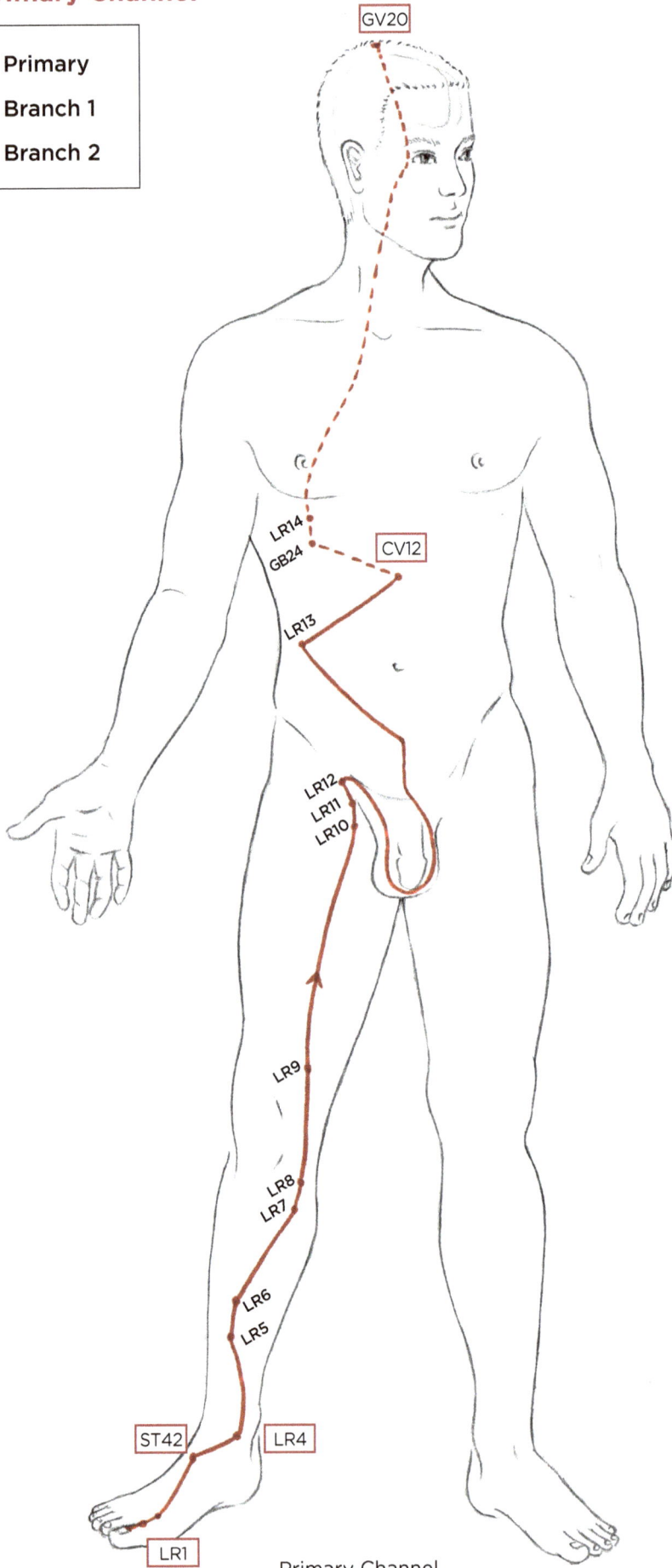

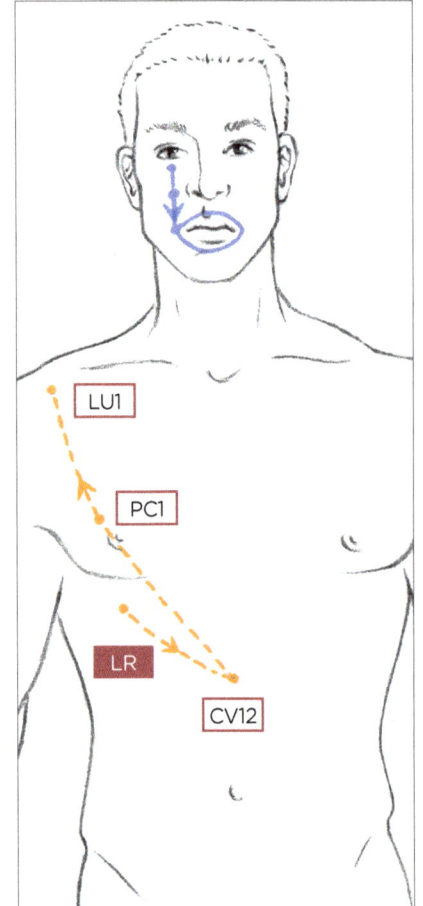

Legend:
- Primary
- Branch 1
- Branch 2

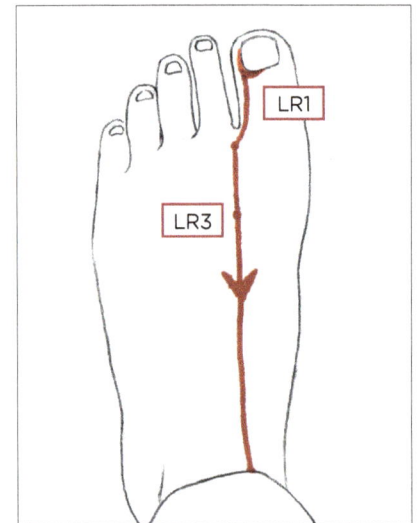

GV20

LR14
GB24
CV12
LR13
LR12
LR11
LR10
LR9
LR8
LR7
LR6
LR5
ST42
LR4
LR1

Primary Channel

LU1
PC1
LR
CV12

Branch 1
Branch 2

LR1
LR3

Primary - detail

Point Location
Guide

Point Location Reminders

This section is simply a guide to trigger memory of the location of points and assumes that detailed study of an excellent point location text has already occurred. For the study of beautifully presented, individual point drawings and textbook locations, I highly recommend Peter Deadman's, book, flash cards or app of *A Manual of Acupuncture*.

Remember that the textbook location of a point, though necessarily presented and learned with exactness, is merely a guide, often an approximation of the point's location on an individual body. Palpation is key to locating a point in living anatomy.

Unless otherwise stated, points are in depressions, big and small.
C- T- and L- stand for the tips of the spinous processes of the cervical, thoracic and lumbar vertebrae.

* Indicates the point lies over the ribcage and must be needled obliquely, (never perpendicularly). Points on the sternum should also be needled obliquely.

Color code:

■ = Sinew Channel point

■ = Luo point

■ = Divergent Channel point

■ = Eight Extra Channel point

POINT		LOCATION
LU-1	■	6 cun lateral to midline, over the 1st intercostal space. Find the triangular depression under the clavicle about 6 cun lateral to the midline (LU-2). LU-1 is one cun below that and slightly lateral to it. *
LU-2		6 cun lateral to midline, just below the clavicle in a depression medial to the coracoid process.*
LU-3		3 cun below axilla fold, lateral to tendon (biceps).
LU-4		1 cun inferior to LU-3
LU-5		In elbow crease, radial to tendon.
LU-6		7 cun proximal to LU-9
LU-7	■ ■	1.5 cun proximal to LI-5, in a crevice, neither anterior nor posterior, in a tight, narrow notch.
LU-8		1 cun proximal to LU-9.
LU-9		At the wrist crease, in the depression just lateral to the pulse and medial to abductor pollicis longus.

LU-10		At the midpoint of the first metacarpal, between the bone and the fleshiness of the thenar eminence.
LU-11	🟧	Anywhere close to the thumb cuticle that appears slightly irritated after you hold firmly the end of the thumb and nail.
LI-1	🟧	Anywhere close to the index finger cuticle that appears slightly irritated after you hold firmly the end of the finger and nail.
LI-2		On the radial edge of the index finger, close to the metacarpophalangeal joint.
LI-3		On the radial edge of the palm, 1.25 cun proximal to LI-2.
LI-4		Radial to the midpoint of the second metacarpal.
LI-5		On the radial edge of the wrist, in a depression found when the thumb is fully extended. Relax the thumb before needling.
LI-6	🟥	3 cun proximal to LI-5 on a line between LI-5 and LI-11, in a wide, diagonal dish-like depression bound by bands.
LI-7		5 cun proximal to LI-5 (on the LI-5 to LI-11 line).
LI-8		7 cun proximal to LI-5 (on the LI-5 to LI-11 line).
LI-9		9 cun proximal to LI-5 (on the LI-5 to LI-11 line).
LI-10		10 cun proximal to LI-5 (on the LI-5 to LI-11 line).
LI-11		At the lateral end of the elbow crease when the elbow is bent.
LI-12		1 cun lateral and superior to LI-11.
LI-13		3 cun proximal to LI-11 on a line between LI-11 and LI-15.
LI-14	🟦	In the depression between deltoid and brachialis on the line between LI-11 and LI-15.
LI-15	🟩🟦	In a depression anterior and inferior to the acromion on the edge of the shoulder, at the very top of the arm. Find the notch and needle down the arm.

🟧 🟥	Sinew, Luo
🟩 🟦	Divergent, 8X

LI-16	🟦	At the lateral end of the depression between the scapula spine and the clavicle. Lay the needle almost flat and needle very obliquely away from the shoulder. ✻
LI-17		At the posterior border of the sternocleidomastoid (SCM) muscle, 1 cun inferior to the level of the cricoid cartilage.
LI-18	🟩	Between the heads of SCM at the level of the cricoid cartilage. Needle obliquely, downward and slightly medially, in line with the SCM.
LI-19		Inferior to the lateral interior of the nostril, a third of the distance between the nose and lip.
LI-20	🟩	In the groove at the side of the nose at the midpoint of the roundness of the side of the nose.
ST-1	🟦	Between the eye and infraorbital ridge, below the pupil. Needle very superficially, lay the needle flat.
ST-2		1 cun inferior to ST-1
ST-3	🟧🟦	Below the pupil, level with the rounded fleshy part of the nose.
ST-4	🟩🟦	0.4 cun lateral to the corner of the mouth. Use a half inch needle.
ST-5	🟩	Anterior to the angle of the mandible, at the anterior border of the masseter muscle. Needle inferiorly.
ST-6		About 1 cun superior and anterior to the angle of the mandible between the heads of masseter muscle. Needle toward the mandible angle.
ST-7		On the inferior edge of the zygomatic arch, anterior to the mandible.
ST-8	🟧	4.5 cun lateral to the midline and 0.5 cun within the hairline, in a notch.
ST-9	🟩🟦	At the level of the cricoid cartilage, between that cartilage and the carotid artery. Find the beating carotid and needle just medial to it, perpendicularly.

🟧🟥	Sinew, Luo
🟩🟦	Divergent, 8X

ST-10		Midway between ST-9 and ST-11.
ST-11		Just superior to the clavicle between the heads of SCM.
ST-12	🟩🟦	In the supraclavicular fossa, 4 cun lateral to the midline. Lay your needle almost flat and skirt the clavicle. Never perpendicular. *
ST-13		Directly inferior to ST-12 on the inferior border of the clavicle. *
ST-14		4 cun lateral to the midline at the first intercostal space. *
ST-15	🟩	4 cun lateral to the midline at the second intercostal space. *
ST-16		4 cun lateral to the midline at the third intercostal space. *
ST-17		The nipple. For location reference only. No treatment. *
ST-18		4 cun lateral to the midline at the fifth intercostal space. *
ST-19		2 cun lateral to the midline, 6 cun superior to umbilicus. *
ST-20		2 cun lateral to the midline, 5 cun superior to umbilicus.
ST-21		2 cun lateral to the midline, 4 cun superior to umbilicus.
ST-22		2 cun lateral to the midline, 3 cun superior to umbilicus.
ST-23		2 cun lateral to the midline, 2 cun superior to umbilicus.
ST-24		2 cun lateral to the midline, 1 cun superior to umbilicus.
ST-25		2 cun lateral to the umbilicus.
ST-26	🟩🟦	2 cun lateral to the midline, 1 cun inferior to umbilicus.
ST-27		2 cun lateral to the midline, 2 cun inferior to umbilicus.
ST-28		2 cun lateral to the midline, 3 cun inferior to umbilicus. *
ST-29		2 cun lateral to the midline, 4 cun inferior to umbilicus. *
ST-30	🟩🟦	2 cun lateral to the midline, level with CV-2 which is at the superior edge of the pubic symphysis. *

🟧🟥	Sinew, Luo
🟩🟦	Divergent, 8X

85

ST-31		Imagine a line between the ASIS and the lateral patella. Imagine another line across the body level with two 2 cun below CV-2. ST-31 is where these two lines meet, lateral to sartorius.
ST-32		6 cun superior to the patella on the ASIS to lateral patella line.
ST-33		3 cun superior to the patella on the ASIS to lateral patella line.
ST-34		2 cun superior to the patella on the ASIS to lateral patella line.
ST-35		At the lateral eye of the knee (inferior to the patella, lateral to its ligament).
ST-36	🟦	3 cun inferior to ST-35, one finger's breadth lateral to the most anterior aspect of the tibia. Closer to the tibia than you might think.
ST-37	🟦	3 cun inferior to ST-36, one finger's breadth lateral to the most anterior aspect of the tibia.
ST-38		2 cun inferior to ST-37, one finger's breadth lateral to the most anterior aspect of the tibia. (8 cun superior to the lateral malleolus.)
ST-39	🟦	1 cun inferior to ST-38, one finger's breadth lateral to the most anterior aspect of the tibia. (7 cun superior to the lateral malleolus.)
ST-40	🟥	8 cun superior to the lateral malleolus, two fingers' breadth lateral to the most anterior aspect of the tibia. It's in a shallow dish-like depression.
ST-41		Level with the medial malleolus in a hollow in the center of the anterior ankle between the two extensor tendons.
ST-42	🟦	The point is at the dorsalis pedis artery pulse 1.5 cun distal to ST-41, where four bones meet (cuneiforms 2 and 3 and metatarsals 2 and 3). Sometimes I find this difficult and end up a little more distal than that. It works just as beautifully.
ST-43		Between the second and third metatarsals, 1 cun proximal to the web.
ST-44		On the web, 0.5 cun proximal from its distal border.
ST-45	🟧	Anywhere close to the fourth toe cuticle that appears slightly irritated after you hold firmly the end of the toe and nail.

🟧 🟥	Sinew, Luo
🟩 🟦	Divergent, 8X

SP-1	🟧🟦	Anywhere close to the big toe cuticle that appears slightly irritated after you hold firmly the end of the toe and nail.
SP-2		On the medial side of the big toe, just distal and slightly inferior to the metatarsophalangeal joint.
SP-3		Proximal and inferior to the first metatarsophalangeal joint.
SP-4	🟥🟦	Find the base of the first metatarsal which feels like a protrusion and then press and slide your finger distally and inferiorly until you fall into a slight, often tightly bound depression.
SP-5		Put your finger on the tip of the medial malleolus and slide it distally and inferiorly to fall into a depression.
SP-6		3 cun superior to the medial malleolus, just posterior to the tibia.
SP-7		6 cun superior to the medial malleolus, just posterior to the tibia.
SP-8		Find SP-9, press and slide your finger distally 3 cun where it sinks into a slight depression.
SP-9		In a major depression posterior and inferior to the medial condyle of the tibia.
SP-10		2 cun above the patella, level with its medial edge.
SP-11		6 cun proximal to SP-10 on the line connecting SP-10 and SP-12.
SP-12	🟩🟦	In a depression 3.5 cun lateral to CV-2 which is on the midline at the superior border of the pubic symphysis. If you have difficulty finding this point, go a little more lateral. Needle obliquely, inferiorly and slightly medially, parallel to the line of the inguinal crease.
SP-13	🟦	4 cun lateral to the midline, less than 1 cun superior to the level of CV-2.
SP-14		4 cun lateral to the midline, 1.3 cun below the level of the umbilicus.
SP-15	🟩🟦	4 cun lateral to umbilicus.

🟧🟥	Sinew, Luo
🟩🟦	Divergent, 8X

SP-16	■	4 cun lateral to the midline, 3 cun above SP-15.*
SP-17, 18, 19, 20		6 cun lateral to midline, over the 5th, 4th, 3rd and 2nd intercostal spaces respectively. *
SP-21	■ ■	On the lateral midline, 6 cun below the axilla in the 6th intercostal space. *
HT-1	■	In a depression at the center of the axilla. Needle superiorly, never toward the chest. *
HT-2		3 cun proximal to HT-3.
HT-3		At the medial end of the elbow crease when the arm is flexed.
HT-4		1.5 cun proximal to HT-7, on the radial side of the tendon.
HT-5	■	1 cun proximal to HT-7, on the radial side of the tendon.
HT-6		0.5 cun proximal to HT-7, on the radial side of the tendon.
HT-7		At the proximal border of the pisiform bone, on the radial side of the tendon.
HT-8		Where the little finger touches the palm when making a fist.
HT-9	■	Anywhere at all close to the little finger cuticle that appears slightly irritated after you hold firmly the end of the finger and nail.
SI-1	■	Anywhere at all close to the little finger cuticle that appears slightly irritated after you hold firmly the end of the finger and nail.
SI-2		On the ulnar border of the little finger, close to the metacarpophalangeal joint.
SI-3	■	On the ulnar border of the hand, in the depression proximal to the metacarpophalangeal joint.
SI-4		On the ulnar border of the hand, just distal to the triquetral bone.
SI-5		On the ulnar border of the wrist, just distal to the head of the ulna.

■ ■	Sinew, Luo
■ ■	Divergent, 8X

SI-6		In the depression medial to the head of the ulna.
SI-7	🟥	In a tiny dip which feels like an irregularity in the muscle when pressing through it to the bone, 5 cun proximal to SI-5 on a line between SI-5 and SI-8.
SI-8		In the bony depression medial to the tip of the elbow.
SI-9		1 cun superior to the posterior end of the axillary crease.
SI-10	🟩🟦	Just inferior to the spine of the scapula, directly superior to the end of the axillary crease.
SI-11		In the most tender spot in the central area of the scapula.
SI-12		Superior to the midpoint of the spine of the scapula.
SI-13		Midway between SI-10 and T2.
SI-14		3 cun lateral to T1. *
SI-15		2 cun lateral to C7.
SI-16		On the posterior border of SCM lateral to ST-9 and LI-18.
SI-17		Between the angle of the mandible and SCM.
SI-18	🟧🟩	Just under the cheekbone, directly inferior to the outer canthus of the eye.
SI-19		In front of the ear, between the middle of the tragus and the mandible.
BL-1	🟩🟦	In the depression just superior to the inner canthus of the eye. Use a half inch needle and needle perpendicularly.
BL-2		Directly superior to the inner canthus on the eyebrow.
BL-3		0.5 cun superior to the hairline, directly superior to BL-1.
BL-4		0.5 cun superior to the hairline, 1.5 cun lateral to the midline.
BL-5		1 cun superior to the hairline, 1.5 cun lateral to the midline.

🟧🟥	Sinew, Luo
🟩🟦	Divergent, 8X

BL-6		2.5 cun superior to the hairline, 1.5 cun lateral to the midline.
BL-7		4 cun back from the anterior hairline, 1.5 cun lateral to the midline.
BL-8		5.5 cun back from the anterior hairline, 1.5 cun lateral to the midline.
BL-9		Find the occipital protuberance, and go 1.25 cun lateral.
BL-10	🟩	In the big depression created under the occiput, just lateral to trapezius.
		Note that the Bladder Shu points, when used in Divergent Channels are 0.5 cun lateral to the midline. (Hua To points.)
BL-11		1.5 cun lateral to the tip of T1.＊ *Influential point of Bone.*
BL-12		1.5 cun lateral to the tip of T2.＊
BL-13		1.5 cun lateral to the tip of T3.＊ *Lung Shu point.*
BL-14		1.5 cun lateral to the tip of T4.＊ *Pericardium Shu point.*
BL-15	🟩	1.5 cun lateral to the tip of T5.＊ *Heart Shu point.*
BL-16		1.5 cun lateral to the tip of T6.＊ *Governor Vessel Shu.*
BL-17	🟦	1.5 cun lateral to the tip of T7.＊ *Influential point of Blood and of the Diaphragm.*
BL-18		1.5 cun lateral to the tip of T9.＊ *Liver Shu point.*
BL-19		1.5 cun lateral to the tip of T10.＊ *Gallbladder Shu point.*
BL-20		1.5 cun lateral to the tip of T11.＊ *Spleen Shu point.*
BL-21		1.5 cun lateral to the tip of T12.＊ *Stomach Shu point.*
BL-22		1.5 cun lateral to the tip of L1. *Triple Heater Shu point.*
BL-23	🟩🟦	1.5 cun lateral to the tip of L2. *Kidney Shu point.*

🟧🟥	Sinew, Luo
🟩🟦	Divergent, 8X

BL-24		1.5 cun lateral to the tip of L3.
BL-25		1.5 cun lateral to the tip of L4. *Large Intestine Shu.*
BL-26		1.5 cun lateral to the tip of L5.
BL-27		1.5 cun lateral to the midline, level with the first sacral foramen. *Small Intestine Shu.*
BL-28	🟩	1.5 cun lateral to the midline, level with the second sacral foramen. *Bladder Shu.*
BL-29		1.5 cun lateral to the midline, level with the third sacral foramen.
BL-30		1.5 cun lateral to the midline, level with the fourth sacral foramen.
BL-31		At the first sacral foramen.
BL-32	🟩	At the second sacral foramen.
BL-33		At the third sacral foramen.
BL-34		At the fourth sacral foramen.
BL-35	🟦	0.5 cun lateral to the tip of the coccyx.
BL-36	🟩	Just under the buttock near the midpoint of the leg, in a depression between the hamstring muscles.
BL-37		On the midpoint of the leg, 8 cun superior to BL-40.
BL-38		1 cun superior to BL-39, just medial to biceps femoris.
BL-39		On the popliteal crease, just medial to biceps femoris.
BL-40	🟩🟦	In a depression at the center of the back of the knee, on the popliteal crease.
BL-41		3 cun lateral to the tip of T2.
BL-42		3 cun lateral to the tip of T3.
BL-43		3 cun lateral to the tip of T4.

🟧	🟥	Sinew, Luo
🟩	🟦	Divergent, 8X

BL-44	🟩	3 cun lateral to the tip of T5.
BL-45		3 cun lateral to the tip of T6.
BL-46		3 cun lateral to the tip of T7.
BL-47		3 cun lateral to the tip of T9.
BL-48		3 cun lateral to the tip of T10.
BL-49		3 cun lateral to the tip of T11.
BL-50		3 cun lateral to the tip of T12.
BL-51		3 cun lateral to the tip of L1.
BL-52	🟦	3 cun lateral to the tip of L2.
BL-53		3 cun lateral to the midline, nearly level with the second sacral foramen.
BL-54		3 cun lateral to the midline, level with the superior aspect of the coccyx.
BL-55		2 cun inferior to the center of the back of the knee, on the midline of the leg.
BL-56		5 cun inferior to the center of the back of the knee, on the midline of the leg.
BL-57		8 cun inferior to BL-40, that is, half way from the crease at the knee to the level of the lateral malleolus.
BL-58	🟥	Put your finger on BL-60 and slide straight up the leg 7 cun until you sink into a large soft depression.
BL-59	🟦	3 cun superior to BL-60.
BL-60		In the very large depression posterior to the lateral malleolus.
BL-61	🟦	1.5 cun inferior to BL-60.

🟧	🟥	Sinew, Luo
🟩	🟦	Divergent, 8X

BL-62	▪	1 cun inferior to the prominence of the lateral malleolus.
BL-63	▪	In the large depression posterior to the tuberosity of the fifth metatarsal.
BL-64		Just anterior to the tuberosity of the fifth metatarsal.
BL-65		Just posterior to the head of the fifth metatarsal.
BL-66		On the little toe, just anterior to the metatarsophalangeal joint.
BL-67	▪	Anywhere at all close to the little toe cuticle that appears slightly irritated after you hold firmly the end of the toe.
KI Prime	▪	On the sole of the foot, directly inferior to the medial malleous.
KI-1	▪	In the depression on the sole of the foot, about 2.5 cun posterior to the base of the second toe.
KI-2	▪	Just inferior to the navicular tuberosity.
KI-3		In the very large depression posterior to the medial malleolus.
KI-4	▪	KI-4 in a moon-shaped depression against the tendon, 0.5 cun inferior and to KI-3.
KI-5		1 cun inferior to KI-3.
KI-6	▪	1 cun inferior to the prominence of the medial malleolus between the ligaments there.
KI-7		2 cun superior to KI-3, at the border of the tendon.
KI-8	▪	2 cun superior and 0.5 cun anterior to KI-3.
KI-9	▪	Find LR-5 which is 5 cun proximal to the medial malleolus in a dip in the bone, and slide your finger directly posterior to a soft depression on the Kidney channel.
KI-10	▪ ▪	Between the two tendons at the medial end of the popliteal crease. Needle between the tendons and point the needle inferiorly.

▪ ▪	Sinew, Luo
▪ ▪	Divergent, 8X

KI-11		0.5 cun lateral to CV-2.
KI-12		1 cun superior to KI-11.
KI-13		2 cun superior to KI-11.
KI-14		3 cun superior to KI-11.
KI-15		4 cun superior to KI-11.
KI-16		0.5 cun lateral to the umbilicus.
KI-17		2 cun superior to KI-16.
KI-18		3 cun superior to KI-16.
KI-19		4 cun superior to KI-16.
KI-20		5 cun superior to KI-16.
KI-21		6 cun superior to KI-16.
KI-22		2 cun lateral to the midline in the 5th intercostal space. *
KI-23		2 cun lateral to the midline in the 4th intercostal space, level with the nipple. *
KI-24		2 cun lateral to the midline in the 3rd intercostal space. *
KI-25		2 cun lateral to the midline in the 2nd intercostal space. *
KI-26		2 cun lateral to the midline in the 1st intercostal space. *
KI-27		2 cun lateral to the midline, just beneath the clavicle. *
PC-1		1 cun lateral and superior to the nipple. If you'd rather not needle this point, use GB-22 instead. *

	Sinew, Luo
	Divergent, 8X

PC-2		2 cun inferior to the axillary crease, between the heads of biceps brachii.
PC-3		On the cubital crease, medial to the aponeurosis.
PC-4		5 cun proximal to PC-7.
PC-5		3 cun proximal to PC-7.
PC-6	🟥🟦	2 cun proximal to PC-7, between the tendons where the tendons are most springy. Cradle the wrist in your hand and needle very obliquely toward PC-7.
PC-7		On the midline of the wrist crease, between the tendons.
PC-8		Make a fist. PC-8 is where your middle finger strikes the palm.
PC-9	🟨	At the tip of the middle finger.
TH-1	🟨	Anywhere at all close to the fourth finger cuticle that appears slightly irritated after you hold firmly the end of the finger and nail.
TH-2		At the center of the webbing between the fourth and fifth fingers.
TH-3		1 cun proximal to TH-2.
TH-4		On the dorsal aspect of the wrist, 1 cun distal to SI-6.
TH-5	🟥🟦	2 cun proximal to the dorsal wrist crease, in a round depression, Be sure to be radial to the communis tendon.
TH-6		3 cun proximal to TH-4 between radius and ulna, radial to extensor digitorum communis.
TH-7		3 cun proximal to TH-4 between the ulna and extensor digitorum communis.
TH-8		4 cun proximal to TH-4 between radius and ulna, radial to extensor digitorum communis.
TH-9		7 cun proximal to TH-4, between the radius and the ulna.
TH-10		1 cun proximal to the point of the elbow.

🟨 🟥	Sinew, Luo
🟩 🟦	Divergent, 8X

TH-11		2 cun proximal to the point of the elbow.
TH-12		4 cun proximal to the point of the elbow.
TH-13	■	Two thirds of the distance from TH-10 to TH-14.
TH-14	■	Put two fingers in the depressions on either side of the end of the acromion at the very top of the arm. The anterior finger is in LI-15 and the posterior finger is in TH-14.
TH-15	■	1 cun posterior to GB-21. *
TH-16	■	1 cun inferior to the depression at the mastoid process, on the posterior border of SCM.
TH-17		Between the mandible and the mastoid process.
TH-18		1.5 cun posterior and superior to TH-17, on the mastoid bone.
TH-19		1.25 cun superior to TH-18, on the mastoid bone.
TH-20		On the head, level with the highest point of the ear.
TH-21		In the groove superior to the mandible just anterior to the ear.
TH-22		0.5 cun anterior to the superior border of where the ear and head meet.
TH-23		At the lateral end of the eyebrow.
GB-1	■	0.5 cun lateral to the outer canthus. This point is close to the eye. Be sure to be medial to the (most often not visible) blood vessel that is about 0.7 cun from the canthus. Use a half inch needle pointed toward the eye with very shallow insertion, anchoring your hand gently on the patient. Assure the patient it is a very shallow insertion.
GB-2		Between the inferior tragic notch and the mandible.
GB-3		Superior to ST-7, superior to the zygomatic arch.
GB-4		1 cun inferior to ST-8

■	■	Sinew, Luo
■	■	Divergent, 8X

GB-5		Half way between ST-8 and GB-7.
GB-6		1 cun superior and slightly anterior to GB-7.
GB-7		One finger's breadth anterior to the highest point of the ear.
GB-8	🟩	1 cun superior to the highest point of the ear.
GB-9		0.5 cun posterior to GB-8.
GB-10		1 cun inferior and posterior to GB-9.
GB-11		1.5 cun inferior GB-10.
GB-12	🟩	At the depression posterior to the mastoid process.
GB-13	🟧🟦	0.5 cun posterior to the hairline, 3 cun lateral to the midline.
GB-14		1 cun superior to the middle of each eyebrow.
GB-15	🟦	0.5 cun superior to the hairline, halfway between the midline and ST-8.
GB-16	🟦	1.5 cun posterior to GB-15.
GB-17	🟦	3 cun posterior to GB-15.
GB-18	🟦	4.5 cun posterior to GB-15.
GB-19	🟦	1.5 cun superior to GB-20.
GB-20	🟦	In the large depression at the base of the skull, midway between the midline and GB-12. Needle inferiorly.
GB-21	🟦	At the highest point of the shoulder, directly superior to the angle of the scapula.*
GB-22	🟧🟥🟩🟦	3 cun inferior to the axilla on the lateral midline between two ribs that are very close together, level with the nipple.* The Great Luo of the Spleen. Needle very obliquely, parallel to the ribs.

🟧🟥	Sinew, Luo
🟩🟦	Divergent, 8X

GB-23		1 cun anterior to GB-22.*
GB-24	🟩	4 cun lateral to the midline at the 7th intercostal space.*
GB-25	🟩	At the end of the 12th rib.*
GB-26	🟩🟦	On the lateral midline, level with the umbilicus.
GB-27	🟦	Just anterior to the anterior superior iliac spine.
GB-28	🟦	0.5 cun anterior and inferior to GB-27.
GB-29	🟦	Midway between the ASIS and the greater trochanter.
GB-30	🟩	In the deepest depression in the buttock, a third of the distance from the greater trochanter to the superior aspect of the coccyx.
GB-31		On the lateral midline of the thigh where the patient's middle finger reaches. (About 7 cun superior to the knee crease.)
GB-32		2 cun inferior to GB-31.
GB-33		On the lateral midline, level with the superior aspect of the patella.
GB-34		1 cun anterior and inferior to the head of the fibula, about 4 cun inferior to GB-33.
GB-35	🟦	7 cun superior to the tip of the lateral malleolus, just posterior to the fibula.
GB-36		7 cun superior to the tip of the lateral malleolus, just anterior to the fibula.
GB-37	🟥	GB-37 in a significant depression 5 cun superior to the tip of the lateral malleolus, just anterior to the fibula.
GB-38		4 cun superior to the tip of the lateral malleolus, just anterior to the fibula.
GB-39		3 cun superior to the tip of the lateral malleolus, just posterior to the fibula.

🟧	🟥	Sinew, Luo
🟩	🟦	Divergent, 8X

GB-40		Just anterior and inferior to the lateral malleolus.
GB-41	🟦	Between the tendon that branches to the little toe and the fifth metatarsal.
GB-42		Between the fourth and fifth metatarsals and just proximal to their heads, medial to the tendon that branches to the little toe.
GB-43		In the middle of the webbing between the fourth and fifth toes.
GB-44	🟧	Anywhere at all close to the fourth toe cuticle that appears slightly irritated after you hold firmly the end of the toe and nail.

LR-1	🟧🟦	Anywhere at all close to the big toe cuticle that appears slightly irritated after you hold firmly the end of the toe and nail.
LR-2		In the middle of the webbing between the big and second toes.
LR-3		In the big depression between the first and second metatarsals.
LR-4		Between the medial malleolus and the tibialis anterior tendon.
LR-5	🟥🟩	5 cun superior to the medial malleolus, in a significant notch in the medial face of the tibia.
LR-6		7 cun proximal to the medial malleolus, between the tibia and gastrocnemius.
LR-7		1 cun posterior to SP-9.
LR-8		Just superior to the medial end of the knee crease, anterior to the tendons, in the loosest part of that depression.
LR-9		4 cun superior to LR-8.
LR-10		3 cun inferior to ST-30.
LR-11		2 cun inferior to ST-30.
LR-12		1 cun inferior and 2.5 cun lateral to CV-2.
LR-13	🟩🟦	Just inferior and anterior to the end of the 11th rib.*

🟧 🟥	Sinew, Luo
🟩 🟦	Divergent, 8X

LR-14	🟩🟦	4 cun lateral to the midline, in the 6th intercostal space.*
CV-1	🟦	In the center of the perineum.
CV-2	🟩🟦	On the midline on the superior border of the pubic bone.
CV-3	🟧🟩🟦	4 cun inferior to the umbilicus. *Bladder Mu point.*
CV-4	🟩🟦	3 cun inferior to the umbilicus. *Small Intestine Mu point.*
CV-5	🟦	2 cun inferior to the umbilicus. *Triple Heater Mu point.*
CV-6	🟦	1.5 cun inferior to the umbilicus.
CV-7	🟦	1 cun inferior to the umbilicus.
CV-8	🟩🟦	In the center of the umbilicus.
CV-9	🟦	1 cun superior to the umbilicus.
CV-10	🟦	2 cun superior to the umbilicus.
CV-11	🟦	3 cun superior to the umbilicus.
CV-12	🟩🟦	4 cun superior to the umbilicus. *Stomach Mu point.*
CV-13	🟦	5 cun superior to the umbilicus.
CV-14	🟩🟦	6 cun superior to the umbilicus. *Heart Mu point.*
CV-15	🟧🟦	CV-15 in a depression immediately inferior to the base of the xyphoid. *Luo point of Ren Mai.*
CV-16	🟦	At the junction of the sternum and the xyphoid process.*
CV-17	🟩🟦	On the sternum, level with the nipple.*

🟧 🟥	Sinew, Luo
🟩 🟦	Divergent, 8X

CV-18	▪	On the sternum, level with the third intercostal space.＊
CV-19	▪	On the sternum, level with the second intercostal space.＊
CV-20	▪	On the sternum, level with the first intercostal space.＊
CV-21	▪	On the sternum about 1 cun inferior to CV-22.＊
CV-22	▪▪	0.5 cun superior to the sternum.
CV-23	▪▪	In the depression superior to the hyoid bone.
CV-24	▪	In the deepest depression between the bottom lip and the chin.
GV-1	▪▪	In a depression immediately inferior to the base of the coccyx.
GV-2	▪	Between the sacrum and the coccyx.
GV-3	▪	Just beneath the tip of L4.
GV-4	▪▪	Just beneath the tip of L2.
GV-5	▪	Just beneath the tip of L1.
GV-6	▪	Just beneath the tip of T11.
GV-7	▪	Just beneath the tip of T10.
GV-8	▪	Just beneath the tip of T9.
GV-9	▪	Just beneath the tip of T7.
GV-10	▪	Just beneath the tip of T6.
GV-11	▪▪	Just beneath the tip of T5.
GV-12	▪	Just beneath the tip of T3.

▪▪	Sinew, Luo
▪▪	Divergent, 8X

GV-13	🟦	Just beneath the tip of T1.
GV-14	🟩🟦	Just beneath the tip of C7.
GV-15	🟦	0.5 cun inferior to GV-16.
GV-16	🟦	Just inferior to the occipital protuberance.
GV-17	🟦	1.5 cun superior to GV-16.
GV-18	🟦	1.5 cun superior to GV-17.
GV-19	🟦	1.5 cun superior to GV-18. Also 1.5 cun posterior to GV-20.
GV-20	🟩🟦	At the crown, where hair grows in different directions, 5 cun from the anterior hairline and 7 cun from the posterior hairline.
GV-21	🟦	1.5 cun anterior to GV-20, 3.5 cun posterior to the front hairline.
GV-22	🟦	2 cun posterior to the front hairline.
GV-23	🟦	1 cun posterior to the front hairline.
GV-24	🟦	0.5 cun posterior to the front hairline.
GV-25	🟦	At the tip of the nose.
GV-26	🟦	One third of the distance from the nose to the upper lip.
GV-27	🟦	At the meeting of the upper lip and the philtrum.
GV-28	🟦	Inside the mouth where the upper lip and the gum meet.

🟧🟥	Sinew, Luo
🟩🟦	Divergent, 8X

www.ingramcontent.com/pod-product-compliance
Lightning Source LLC
Chambersburg PA
CBHW041427270326
41932CB00030B/3487